Perinatal HIV

What health professionals need to know

Developed by the
Perinatal Education Programme

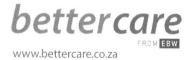

FROM EBW

www.bettercare.co.za

VERY IMPORTANT

We have taken every care to ensure that drug dosages and related medical advice in this book are accurate. However, drug dosages can change and are updated often, so always double-check dosages and procedures against a reliable, up-to-date formulary and the given drug's documentation before administering it.

Perinatal HIV:
What health professionals need to know

Updated 31 March 2014

Layout updated 1 August 2011

Updated 7 May 2010

First published in manual format by the Perinatal Education Programme in 1999

Revised and republished by Bettercare in 2008

Text © Perinatal Education Programme 2008

Getup © Electric Book Works 2008

ISBN (paperback): 978-1-920218-20-1

ISBN (PDF ebook): 978-1-920218-58-4

Visit our websites www.electricbookworks.com and www.bettercare.co.za

Contents

Acknowledgements

The aim of this Perinatal HIV course is to improve the care of HIV-positive pregnant women and their newborn infants in all communities, especially in poor peri-urban and rural districts of southern Africa.

Perinatal HIV was developed by a multi-disciplinary team of nurses, obstetricians, paediatricians, senior professors and colleagues in government health departments. This ensures a balanced, practical and up-to-date approach to common and important clinical problems.

We acknowledge the contributions of the following colleagues, each an expert in their own field of perinatal care or HIV management:

Prof M. Adhikari; Dr R. Bobat; Dr J. Burgess; Sr F. Cope; Dr M. Cotton;

Prof H. de Groot; Dr G. Gray; Dr D. Greenfield; Prof G. Hussey; Sr M. Kreft; Prof G. Maartens; Mrs S. Martindale-Tucker; Dr J. McIntyre; Dr C. Orrell; Sr M. Petersen; Dr K. Pillay; Prof G. Theron

We also acknowledge all the participants of the *Perinatal HIV* course who over the years have made suggestions and offered constructive criticism. It is only through constant feedback from colleagues and participants that the content of our courses can be improved.

We would like to thank Eduhealthcare for funding this publication.

Editor-in-chief of the Perinatal Education Programme, Prof D. L. Woods

Introduction

About the Bettercare series

Bettercare publishes an innovative series of distance-learning books for healthcare professionals, developed by the Perinatal Education Trust, Eduhealthcare, the Desmond Tutu HIV Foundation and the Desmond Tutu TB Centre, with contributions from numerous experts.

Our aim is to provide appropriate, affordable and up-to-date learning material for healthcare workers in under-resourced areas, so that they can manage their own continuing education courses which will enable them to learn, practise and deliver skillful, efficient patient care.

The Bettercare series is built on the experience of the Perinatal Education Programme (PEP), which has provided learning opportunities to over 60 000 nurses and doctors in South Africa since 1992. Many of the educational methods developed by PEP are now being adopted by the World Health Organisation (WHO).

Why decentralised learning?

Continuing education for healthcare workers traditionally consists of courses and workshops run by formal trainers at large central hospitals. These teaching courses are expensive to attend, often far away from the healthcare workers' family and places of work, and the content frequently fails to address the real healthcare requirements of the poor, rural communities who face the biggest healthcare challenges.

To help solve these many problems, a self-help decentralised learning method has been developed which addresses the needs of professional healthcare workers, especially those in poor, rural communities.

Books in the Bettercare series

Maternal Care addresses all the common and important problems that occur during pregnancy, labour, delivery and the puerperium. It covers the antenatal and postnatal care of healthy women with normal pregnancies, monitoring and managing the progress of labour, specific medical problems during pregnancy, labour and the puerperium, family planning and regionalised perinatal care. Skills workshops teach clinical examination in pregnancy and labour, routine screening tests, use of an antenatal card and partogram, measuring blood pressure, detecting proteinuria and performing and repairing an episiotomy.

Maternal Care is aimed at healthcare workers in level 1 hospitals or clinics.

Primary Maternal Care addresses the needs of healthcare workers who provide antenatal and postnatal care, but do not conduct deliveries. It is adapted from theory chapters and skills workshops from *Maternal Care*. This book is ideal for midwives and doctors providing primary maternal care in level 1 district hospitals and clinics, and complements the national protocol of antenatal care in South Africa.

Intrapartum Care was developed for doctors and advanced midwives who care for women who deliver in district hospitals. It contains theory chapters and skills workshops adapted from the labour chapters of *Maternal Care*. Particular attention is given to the care of the mother, the management of labour and monitoring the wellbeing of the fetus. *Intrapartum Care* was written to support and complement the national protocol of intrapartum care in South Africa.

Newborn Care was written for healthcare workers providing special care for newborn infants in regional hospitals. It covers resuscitation at birth, assessing infant size and gestational age, routine care and

feeding of both normal and high-risk infants, the prevention, diagnosis and management of hypothermia, hypoglycaemia, jaundice, respiratory distress, infection, trauma, bleeding and congenital abnormalities, as well as communication with parents. Skills workshops address resuscitation, size measurement, history, examination and clinical notes, nasogastric feeds, intravenous infusions, use of incubators, measuring blood glucose concentration, insertion of an umbilical vein catheter, phototherapy, apnoea monitors and oxygen therapy.

Primary Newborn Care was written specifically for nurses and doctors who provide primary care for newborn infants in level 1 clinics and hospitals. *Primary Newborn Care* addresses the care of infants at birth, care of normal infants, care of low-birth-weight infants, neonatal emergencies, and common minor problems in newborn infants.

Mother and Baby Friendly Care describes gentler, kinder, evidence-based ways of caring for women during pregnancy, labour and delivery. It also presents improved methods of providing infant care with an emphasis on kangaroo mother care and exclusive breastfeeding.

Saving Mothers and Babies was developed in response to the high maternal and perinatal mortality rates found in most developing countries. Learning material used in the book is based on the results of the annual confidential enquiries into maternal deaths and the Saving Mothers and Saving Babies reports published in South Africa. It addresses the basic principles of mortality audit, maternal mortality, perinatal mortality, managing mortality meetings and ways of reducing maternal and perinatal mortality rates. This book should be used together with the Perinatal Problem Identification Programme (PPIP).

Birth Defects was written for healthcare workers who look after individuals with birth defects, their families, and women who are at increased risk of giving birth to an infant with a birth defect. Special attention is given to modes of inheritance, medical genetic counselling, and birth defects due to chromosomal abnormalities, single gene defects, teratogens and multifactorial inheritance. This book is being used in the Genetics Education Programme which trains healthcare workers in genetic counselling in South Africa.

Perinatal HIV enables midwives, nurses and doctors to care for pregnant women and their infants in communities where HIV infection is common. Special emphasis has been placed on the prevention of mother-to-infant transmission of HIV. It covers the basics of HIV infection and screening, antenatal and intrapartum care of women with HIV infection, care of HIV-exposed newborn infants, and parent counselling.

Childhood HIV enables nurses and doctors to care for children with HIV infection. It addresses an introduction to HIV in children, the clinical and immunological diagnosis of HIV infection, management of children with and without antiretroviral treatment, antiretroviral drugs, opportunistic infections and end-of-life care.

Childhood TB was written to enable healthcare workers to learn about the primary care of children with tuberculosis. The book covers an introduction to TB infection, and the clinical presentation, diagnosis, management and prevention of tuberculosis in children and HIV/TB co-infection. *Childhood TB* was developed by paediatricians with wide experience in the care of children with tuberculosis, through the auspices of the Desmond Tutu Tuberculosis Centre at the University of Stellenbosch.

Child Healthcare addresses all the common and important clinical problems in children, including immunisation, history and examination, growth and nutrition, acute and chronic infections, parasites, and skin conditions, as well as difficulties in the home and society. Child Healthcare was developed for use in primary care settings.

Adult HIV covers an introduction to HIV infection, management of HIV-infected adults at primary-care clinics, preparing patients for antiretroviral (ARV) treatment, ARV drugs, starting and maintaining patients on ARV treatment and an approach to opportunistic infections. *Adult HIV* was developed by doctors and nurses with wide experience in the care of adults with HIV, through the auspices of the Desmond Tutu HIV Foundation at the University of Cape Town.

Well Women was written for primary health workers who manage the everyday health needs of women. It covers reproductive health, family planning and infertility, common genital infections, vaginal bleeding, and the abuse of women.

Breast Care was written for nurses and doctors who manage the health needs of women from childhood to old age. It covers the assessment and management of benign breast conditions, breast cancer and palliative care.

Infection Prevention and Control was written for nurses, doctors, and health administrators working in the field of infection prevention and control, particularly in resource-limited settings. It includes chapters on IPC programmes, risk management, health facility design, outbreak surveillance and antimicrobial stewardship.

Format of the courses

1. Objectives
The learning objectives are clearly stated at the start of each chapter. They help the participant to identify and understand the important lessons to be learned.

2. Pre- and post-tests
There is a multiple-choice test of 20 questions for each chapter at the end of the book. Participants are encouraged to take a pre-test before starting each chapter, to benchmark their current knowledge, and a post-test after each chapter, to assess what they have learned.

Self-assessment allows participants to monitor their own progress through the course.

3. Question-and-answer format
Theoretical knowledge is presented in a question-and-answer format, which encourages the learner to actively participate in the learning process. In this way, the participant is led step by step through the definitions, causes, diagnosis, prevention, dangers and management of a particular problem.

Participants should cover the answer for a few minutes with a piece of paper while thinking about the correct reply to each question. This method helps learning.

Simplified flow diagrams are also used, where necessary, to indicate the correct approach to diagnosing or managing a particular problem.

Each question is written in bold, like this, and is identified with the number of the chapter, followed by the number of the question, e.g. 5-23.

4. Important lessons

Important practical lessons are emphasised by placing them in a box like this.

5. Notes

NOTE Additional, non-essential information is provided for interest and given in notes like this. These facts are not used in the case studies or included in the multiple-choice questions.

6. Case studies

Each chapter closes with a few case studies which encourage the participant to consolidate and apply what was learned earlier in the chapter. These studies give the participant an opportunity to see the problem as it usually presents itself in the clinic or hospital. The participant should attempt to answer each question in the case study before reading the correct answer.

7. Practical training

Certain chapters contain skills workshops, which need to be practised by the participants (preferably in groups). The skills workshops, which are often illustrated with line drawings, list essential equipment and present step-by-step instructions on how to perform each task. If participants aren't familiar with a practical skill, they are encouraged to ask an appropriate medical or nursing colleague to demonstrate the clinical skill to them. In this way, senior personnel are encouraged to share their skills with their colleagues.

8. Final examination

On completion of each course, participants can take a 75-question multiple-choice examination when they are ready to.

All the exam questions will be taken from the multiple-choice tests from the book. The content of the skills workshops will not be included in the examination.

Participants need to achieve at least 80% in the examination in order to successfully complete the course. Successful candidates will be emailed a certificate which states that they have successfully completed that course. Bettercare courses are not yet accredited for nurses, but South African doctors can earn CPD points on the successful completion of an examination.

Contributors

The developers of our learning materials are a multi-disciplinary team of nurses, midwives, obstetricians, neonatologists, and general paediatricians. The development and review of all course material is overseen by the Editor-in-Chief, emeritus Professor Dave Woods, a previous head of neonatal medicine at the University of Cape Town who now consults to UNICEF and the WHO.

Perinatal Education Trust

Books developed by the Perinatal Education Programme are provided as cheaply as possible. Writing and updating the programme is both funded and managed on a non-profit basis by the Perinatal Education Trust.

Eduhealthcare

Eduhealthcare is a non-profit organisation based in South Africa. It aims to improve health and wellbeing, especially in poor communities, through affordable education for healthcare workers. To this end it provides financial support for the development and publishing of the Bettercare series.

The Desmond Tutu HIV Foundation

The Desmond Tutu HIV Foundation at the University of Cape Town, South Africa, is a centre of excellence in HIV medicine, building capacity through training and enhancing knowledge through research.

The Desmond Tutu Tuberculosis Centre

The Desmond Tutu Tuberculosis Centre at Stellenbosch University, South Africa, strives to improve the health of vulnerable groups through the education of healthcare workers and community members, and by influencing policy based on research into the epidemiology of childhood tuberculosis, multi-drug-resistant tuberculosis, HIV/TB co-infection and preventing the spread of TB and HIV in southern Africa.

Academic Unit for Infection Prevention and Control

The Academic Unit for Infection Prevention and Control (UIPC) is based at Tygerberg Academic Hospital and Stellenbosch University. It resides under the Division of Community Health at the Faculty of Medicine and Health Sciences. The UIPC is responsible for infection prevention and control services and training in the 1300-bed hospital. It also undertakes research and offers academic training to local and international undergraduate and postgraduate students.

Updating the course material

Bettercare learning materials are regularly updated to keep up with developments and changes in healthcare protocols. Course participants can make important contributions to the continual improvement of Bettercare books by reporting factual or language errors, by identifying sections that are difficult to understand, and by suggesting additions or improvements to the contents. Details of alternative or better forms of management would be particularly appreciated. Please send any comments or suggestions to the Editor-in-Chief, Professor Dave Woods.

Contact information

Bettercare

Website: www.bettercare.co.za
Email: info@bettercare.co.za
Cell: 076 657 0353
Fax: 086 219 8093
Post: 3rd Floor, Sunclare Building, 21 Dreyer Street, Claremont, 7708

Perinatal Education Programme

Editor-in-Chief: Professor Dave Woods
Website: www.pepcourse.co.za
Email: pepcourse@mweb.co.za
Phone/fax: 021 786 5369
Post: Perinatal Education Programme, 70 Dorries Drive, Simon's Town, 7975

Exams

exams@bettercare.co.za

1

Introduction to perinatal HIV

Before you begin this unit, please take the corresponding test at the end of the book to assess your knowledge of the subject matter. You should redo the test after you've worked through the unit, to evaluate what you have learned.

Objectives

When you have completed this unit you should be able to:

- Understand the meaning of HIV infection and AIDS.
- Describe the different ways that HIV can be transmitted.
- List the three phases of HIV infection.
- List the common presentations of HIV infection in adults.
- Describe how HIV infection is diagnosed.
- List the factors which influence the risk of becoming infected with HIV.
- Describe how HIV damages the immune system.
- List the groups of drugs used to treat HIV infection.
- Explain how to prevent HIV infection of staff by needle-stick injuries.

Introduction to HIV

1-1 What is HIV?

HIV, the human immunodeficiency virus, is a virus which infects people for life and causes a severe clinical condition called AIDS. HIV infects cells of the immune system, particularly lymphocytes. HIV infection can be spread from one person to another.

. . . .
HIV causes AIDS.
. . . .

HIV infection is a relatively new condition which was first identified in Paris in 1983. Since then it has spread to almost every country in the world and by 2006 over 40 million people worldwide were infected. The number of HIV infected people dropped to 34 million in 2010. In 26 countries the prevalence of HIV decreased by 50% from 2001 to 2012.

In South Africa the prevalence in the age group 15 to 49 years has remained around 17% since 2008. According to the World Health Organisation (WHO) in 2010 South Africa had 260,000 HIV positive women who delivered 48,000 HIV infected infants due to perinatal mother to child transmission. The prevalence of HIV in pregnant women attending public health antenatal clinics in South Africa remained between 28 and 30% from 2004 through to 2011. The National Committee for Confidential Enquiries into Maternal Deaths (NCCEMD) reported 1360 maternal deaths due to AIDS for the triennium 2008 to 2010.

NOTE Two types of HIV are recognised, HIV1 and HIV2. Most infection in southern Africa is caused by HIV1, which has many subtypes (clades). The important subtype in Africa is subtype C, while subtype A is common in West Africa and B is the most common subtype in the developed world.

HIV probably appeared in humans in the 1950s. It was first transmitted to humans by chimpanzees in central Africa. From here it rapidly spread to all parts of the world, especially the USA, Europe, Asia and other parts of Africa.

1-2 What is a virus?

Viruses are extremely small, very simple organisms which can only exist and multiply by invading and taking control of a plant or animal cell (the host cell). Viruses are responsible for many diseases. Unlike bacteria, they are not killed by antibiotics. Viruses may be divided into many different groups. HIV belongs to a group of viruses known as retroviruses.

1-3 What are retroviruses?

They are a group of viruses which are unique in nature as they have a special enzyme which enables them to introduce their own genes into the nucleus of the host cell. The host cell is then instructed to produce millions of

new copies of the virus. These copies are released into the bloodstream where they can infect other cells. Retroviruses usually cause long periods of silent infection before signs of disease appear.

NOTE Retroviruses contain an RNA genetic code. The enzyme reverse transcriptase allows HIV to make DNA copies of its RNA. The DNA copy is then inserted into the DNA of the nucleus in the host cell. This enables the virus to take over control of the host cell and instruct the host cell to produce huge numbers of new HIV. Only retroviruses have this ability to make a DNA copy of their RNA code. Retroviruses are common and some cause cancers in animals.

HIV is a retrovirus.

1-4 What is AIDS?

AIDS stands for the Acquired Immune Deficiency Syndrome. This is a severe illness caused by advanced HIV infection and may present in many different ways. The symptoms and signs of AIDS are usually due to secondary infections with a number of different organisms. Some secondary infections are due to uncommon organisms not normally seen in HIV-negative people. AIDS is a slow, progressive, incurable disease which is fatal unless correctly treated with antiretroviral (ARV) drugs. AIDS was first recognised among homosexual males in the USA in 1981. The following year it was diagnosed in heterosexual men and women in Africa.

AIDS is a severe illness caused by HIV infection. There is a widespread epidemic of AIDS in Africa.

Most cases of AIDS occur in Africa. The spread of the HIV epidemic is greatest in southern Africa. It is estimated that six million adults and children have HIV infection in South Africa alone.

About six million South Africans are infected with HIV.

1-5 Can you have silent HIV infection?

Yes. A person is usually infected with HIV for many years before developing symptoms and signs of the disease. Therefore, most people infected with HIV are clinically well and have a 'silent' or hidden infection.

The spread of HIV

1-6 How can you become infected with HIV?

The virus may be transmitted from one person to another by:

1. Unprotected heterosexual or homosexual intercourse (horizontal transmission).
2. Crossing from a mother to her fetus or newborn infant (vertical transmission).
3. Using syringes, needles, or blades which are soiled with HIV-infected blood. They may be shared by intravenous drug abusers or not

correctly cleaned and then reused by health workers.
4. Accidental needle-stick injuries in healthcare workers.
5. A blood transfusion with HIV-infected blood or other HIV-infected blood products such as factor VIII in haemophiliacs. This is very rare in South Africa as all blood products are screened for HIV.

There is no evidence that HIV can be spread by mosquitoes, lice or bed bugs. In Africa, HIV is most commonly spread by heterosexual intercourse, especially when there are multiple sex partners.

In Africa, HIV is usually spread by sexual intercourse.

1-7 Can an HIV-infected person who is well transmit the virus?

Yes. HIV is frequently transmitted by people who appear to be clinically well but are infected with HIV. This is the great danger of HIV infection as most infectious people do not know that they have been infected. They are also unaware that they may transmit HIV to another person.

1-8 How may you become infected during sexual intercourse?

By contact with infected body fluids which contain large amounts of HIV, such as:

1. Vaginal discharge and cervical secretions
2. Semen

3.	Blood

The spread of HIV between adults by sexual intercourse is called horizontal transmission.

1-9 Can you become infected with HIV during normal social contact?

No. Family and friends of an HIV-infected person do not become infected except by sexual contact. HIV is not transmitted by close social contact such as touching, holding hands, hugging and social kissing. HIV is also not spread by coughing, sneezing, swimming pools, toilet seats, sharing cooking and eating utensils or by changing a nappy. However, any bleeding, such as nose bleeds, may spread HIV if the blood comes in contact with broken skin or mucosal surfaces.

1-10 What forms of sexual contact may transmit HIV?

In Africa HIV is almost always transmitted by penetrative sexual intercourse. However all forms of oral sexual contact (mouth to vagina or mouth to penis) can also result in infection, although the risk is less. Deep kissing may possibly transmit HIV, especially if mouth ulcers are present. HIV is not present in urine or stool while very little is present in saliva. HIV cannot penetrate intact skin but may infect open sores, cuts and abrasions, or mucous membranes. The thin, friable rectal mucosa is easily damaged during anal intercourse and, thereby, increases the risk of infection. Men who have been circumcised have a lower risk of being infected through sexual intercourse.

NOTE The inner surface of the foreskin is easily crossed by HIV infected lymphocytes. Therefore removal of the foreskin is partially protective against men acquiring HIV infection.

1-11 Is HIV very infectious?

In comparison to other viral illnesses such as hepatitis B, HIV is not very infectious, and repeated exposure to large amounts of virus is usually needed for transmission. People with early and advanced HIV infection are most infectious. Other sexually transmitted diseases and abrasions of the vaginal and cervical epithelium increase the risk of infection. The highest risk of sexual transmission for both men and women is during anal intercourse. Patients on ARV treatment are less infectious.

Within weeks of becoming infected, when HIV levels in the blood are very high, promiscuous people with multiple partners may infect many people.

Diagnosing HIV infection

1-12 How is HIV infection diagnosed?

Usually a blood test is used to screen people for antibodies to HIV and HIV antigens (proteins). Antibodies are produced by the immune system to protect the body against invading organisms, such as viruses. Unfortunately they offer little protection to HIV. The presence of HIV antibodies in an adult, or child older than 18 months, indicates HIV infection.

A number of antibody tests are available to diagnose HIV infection.

1. Combined antibody antigen tests have become the standard laboratory test to detect HIV infection. It is a highly accurate test and is used to screen for HIV infection and for confirming a clinical suspicion of HIV infection. From the time of infection it takes between 14 to 21 days for the test to become positive. Two positive tests, using kits from two different manufacturers on the same blood sample, are needed before a definite diagnosis of HIV infection is made. This is done to make sure that an error has not been made. The antigen included in the combined tests is a HIV protein called the p24 antigen.

2. Rapid tests have been developed to detect HIV antibodies in blood, urine and saliva. The new generation of rapid tests detecting both antibodies and antigens are very accurate and in many places have replaced laboratory tests for screening and confirming HIV infection. Two rapid tests using kits from different manufacturers should be used to diagnose HIV infection. The great benefit of the rapid test is that it can be done on site to give same day results. If the rapid test is negative it is very unlikely that the person has HIV infection. Two positive rapid tests indicate HIV infection. If the first rapid test is positive but the second negative, blood must be taken for laboratory testing.

Two positive laboratory or rapid tests are needed to diagnose HIV infection.

Viral tests, which do not rely on HIV antibodies, can also be used to diagnose HIV infection:

1. DNA from the HIV can be detected, using the polymerase chain reaction (PCR) test. This is a very accurate, but more expensive, test which is used in special circumstances to confirm or exclude infection. For example, in infants where the mother's HIV antibodies may remain for up to 18 months and thereby give a positive result in an infant who is not HIV infected. The PCR test is accurate in infants from six weeks after delivery if they have not been breastfed, or in infants who have been breastfed following complete weaning for six weeks. A positive test indicates that the individual is infected with HIV.

2. The virus can be cultured. This is very expensive.

A positive PCR test in an infant indicates that the infant is infected with HIV.

NOTE The DNA-PCR or the total nucleic acid (DNA and RNA) test is used to diagnose HIV infection while the RNA-PCR is usually used to measure viral load.

The antibody tests may be negative for 2 to 8 weeks and the combined antibody antigen laboratory or rapid screening tests may be negative for 14 to 21 days after infection with HIV. This is known as the window period. During the window period these people are still infectious to others, despite their test being negative. The window period for the PCR test is 11 to 12 days.

Clinical signs of HIV infection

1-13 What acute illness may occur soon after HIV infection?

In response to infection with HIV, the immune system produces antibodies against the virus. Unfortunately these antibodies fail to kill all the HIV and cure the infection. At the time that HIV antibodies appear in the blood (seroconversion) some people develop a flu-like illness which lasts a few days or weeks. This illness starts two to four weeks after infection with HIV and is called acute seroconversion illness (or acute HIV syndrome). It only occurs in about half of HIV-infected individuals.

The usual signs of acute seroconversion illness are:

1. Fever
2. General tiredness
3. Enlarged lymph nodes
4. A measles-like rash
5. Cough or sore throat
6. Oral or genital ulcers

The above signs and symptoms are similar to those found in glandular fever (infectious mononucleosis).

NOTE Some people also develop signs of viral meningitis or encephalitis.

During the first few weeks of HIV infection, large amounts of virus are present in the blood and the person is very infectious to others. HIV is most infectious during the acute seroconversion illness. HIV screening tests may still be negative at this time.

> *Acute seroconversion illness is often the first sign of HIV infection.*

1-14 What is the latent phase of HIV infection?

HIV infection, with or without acute seroconversion illness, is followed by months or years when the person feels well. In adults, this silent, asymptomatic period is usually five to ten years but may last for as long as 15 years before the signs of symptomatic HIV infection appear. In children, the latent phase is much shorter, from a few months to five years. Occasionally, asymptomatic HIV-infected adults may also progress rapidly to symptomatic HIV infection. Generalised lymphadenopathy is common in the latent phase.

HIV infection can, therefore, be divided into three phases:

1. Acute seroconversion illness (which only occurs in 50% of people)
2. The latent, asymptomatic phase when people feel well
3. Symptomatic HIV infection when people are ill

Patients who have signs and symptoms due to HIV infection following the latent phase are said to have symptomatic HIV infection (HIV illness or HIV disease). Only when they become severely ill is the clinical condition called AIDS.

1-15 What clinical signs suggest an adult has symptomatic HIV infection?

The clinical signs of symptomatic HIV infection are largely due to a wide range of infections and cancers, which occur because of the damaged immune system.

Common clinical signs in adults with symptomatic HIV infection are:

- Wasting or unexplained weight loss
- Generalised, non-tender lymphadenopathy
- Chronic fever
- Skin rashes
- Mouth infections
- Chronic watery diarrhoea
- Repeated respiratory infections
- Opportunistic infections
- Cancer, especially Kaposi's sarcoma and lymphoma
- Dementia caused by encephalopathy

NOTE HIV may also cause myelopathy and peripheral neuropathy. Oral hairy leucoplakia is asymptomatic but diagnostic of HIV infection.

HIV infection often presents with weight loss and chronic diarrhoea.

The severity of HIV infection can be graded from 1 to 4 based on clinical symptoms and signs. Grade 4 infection is most severe and is called AIDS.

1-16 What are opportunistic infections?

Opportunistic or HIV-associated infections are infections which

usually do not occur in people with a normally functioning immune system. They are severe, repeated or chronic infections with common bacteria and viruses or infections with uncommon organisms. The organisms causing most opportunistic infections in HIV-positive people are:

1. Common bacteria such as Pneumococcus
2. Candida (which causes oral, oesophageal and tracheobronchial thrush)
3. Tuberculosis
4. Pneumocystis carinii and jiroveci (a parasite causing pneumonia)
5. Cytomegalovirus (CMV)
6. Herpes simplex
7. Varicella (the chickenpox virus which causes herpes zoster)
8. Cryptococcus (a fungus which causes meningitis)
9. Cryptosporidium (causes chronic diarrhoea)

Opportunistic infections are common in HIV-infected people due to their damaged immune systems.

An opportunistic infection, such as tuberculosis, is often the first sign that the patient is infected with HIV. Therefore HIV infection must be suspected and screened for in any person who has severe, chronic, repeated or unusual infections.

1-17 Can AIDS be cured?

At present AIDS is a severe, chronic illness which cannot be cured and has a slowly progressive and fatal outcome without the correct management. However, treatment with ARV drugs can prevent the progression of the disease and improve the quality of life for many years. Without treatment, most AIDS patients will die within two years of the onset of the clinical illness. While the amount of virus in the body can be drastically reduced by ARV drugs, some virus unfortunately remains hidden in the lymphocytes. The aim of HIV management is to keep the person well for as long as possible.

Preventing HIV infection

1-18 How can HIV infection be avoided?

HIV infection can be avoided by:

- Abstaining from sexual intercourse
- Having sexual relations only with people who are HIV negative. In practice this usually means having sex with a single HIV-negative partner.
- Using male or female condoms which reduce the risk of infection
- Male circumcision reduces the risk of HIV infection in males.
- Avoiding drugs given intravenously with unsterile needles and syringes
- Avoiding ritual cutting or scratching of the skin with a shared blade
- The routine screening of donated blood and other blood products
- Reducing the risk of mother-to-child transmission
- Encouraging people to get screened for HIV infection

The 'ABC' of preventing HIV infection is **Abstinence**, **Be faithful** to one HIV-negative partner only, and use a **Condom** if there is any chance that the sexual partner may be HIV positive. Delaying the start of sexual activity and then reducing the number of sexual partners is most important. Having more than one sex partner at a time is dangerous. The only way the HIV epidemic will be controlled is by reducing the number of new infections by practising safe sex and by preventing perinatal mother to child transmission of HIV.

Every effort must be made to reduce the number of new HIV infections.

1-19 Do other sexually transmitted diseases increase the risk of HIV infection?

Yes. The presence of other sexually transmitted diseases increases the risk of HIV infection, especially if these other diseases cause ulcers or mucosal damage. Treatment of these sexually transmitted diseases reduces the risk of the sexual spread of HIV.

1-20 Which sexually transmitted diseases may increase the risk of infection with HIV?

Important examples are:

- Syphilis
- Chancroid
- Herpes simplex
- Gonorrhoea
- Chlamydia

The risk of HIV infection is highest if ulcers are present, as in syphilis, chancroid and herpes.

1-21 Are HIV-infected people always infectious to others?

Yes, although the risk of infection varies widely between individuals. HIV is most infectious in the first weeks of the infection and again in seriously ill people when the signs of AIDS develop. At these times there are large amounts of HIV in the blood (a high viral load). The risk of infection is less during the latent period when smaller amounts of HIV are present in the blood. However, most HIV is still spread during the latent period when many people are unaware that they are infected. It is therefore very important that all sexually active adults know their HIV status.

Patients with a high viral load are most infectious.

NOTE Patients who are asymptomatic and on ARV treatment with a undetectable viral load may not be infectious.

1-22 Is HIV equally common in men and women?

No. During heterosexual intercourse HIV is more infectious to women than to men as HIV-infected semen may remain in the vagina for many hours. Therefore, in most countries where sexual transmission is common, HIV infection is more frequent in women.

In South Africa during 2008 to 2011 the adult prevalence of HIV infection in the age group 15 to 24 years ranged between 12 and 13% for females and 5 and 6% for males.

1-23 How does HIV damage the immune system?

HIV invades and destroys the immune system by damaging the CD4 lymphocytes. These special cells are produced by the thymus and control the functions of the immune system. CD4 lymphocytes are also called helper lymphocytes as they assist other types of lymphocytes. A normally functioning immune system prevents severe infections and the development of malignancies. HIV infection causes a fall in the number of CD4 lymphocytes with the result that the immune system cannot function normally. As a result, the risk of infection and cancer increases.

The CD4 count is a very important way of determining the immunological stage of the HIV infection, by measuring the amount of damage that has been done to the immune system.

NOTE Normally the CD4 count in adults is well above 500 cells/µl (usually about 1000 cells/µl). Signs of AIDS usually appear when the count falls below 200. A CD4 count is needed to assess the amount of suppression of the immune system.

The body also responds by producing antibodies to the HIV. Unfortunately, the antibodies cannot kill all the virus, which is able to hide inside cells.

HIV damages the immune system by attacking and destroying the CD4 lymphocytes.

1-24 How does HIV multiply in human cells?

HIV is a retrovirus which infects human CD4 lymphocytes. Retroviruses invade the nucleus of lymphocytes and instruct these 'host' cells to produce more copies of the virus. HIV therefore 'hijacks' the host cell and converts it into a factory which produces millions of new viruses. Antiretroviral drugs act by stopping the multiplication of HIV in lymphocytes.

Managing HIV infection

1-25 What drugs can be used to treat HIV infection?

There are a number of drugs which can reduce the amount of HIV in the body and, thereby, slow the progression to AIDS, or improve the clinical signs of AIDS. At present none of these drugs can cure AIDS. They are called antiretroviral (ARV) drugs. It is best to use at least three of these drugs together. Combination therapy is more effective and helps to avoid drug resistance.

There are four groups of ARV drugs. They block the function of enzymes needed for the multiplication of HIV.

1. Nucleoside and nucleotide reverse transcriptase inhibitors ('nucs'), such as tenofovir (TDF), zidovudine (AZT), lamivudine (3TC) and emtricitabine (FTC). These drugs stop HIV from infecting cells.

2. Non-nucleoside reverse transcriptase inhibitors ('non-nucs'), such as nevirapine (NVP) and efavirenz (EFV). They also stop HIV from infecting cells.

3. Protease inhibitors ('PIs'), such as ritonavir and lopinavir. These drugs prevent the HIV-infected cell from releasing new virus.

4. Integrase inhibitors, such as raltegravir that block integrase, a viral enzyme that inserts the viral genetic messages into the DNA of the host cell. The drug is available in a limited number of public health facilities in South Africa and is used if HIV acquires resistance to other drugs.

NOTE Other nucleoside reverse transcriptase inhibitors include didanosine (ddi) and stavudine (d4T), while other protease inhibitors include indinavir, saquinavir and nelfinavir. The two groups of reverse transcriptase inhibitors act differently in preventing HIV infection of cells.

ARV drugs can be used to treat a patient with severe HIV infection (ARV treatment) or to prevent infection with HIV (ARV prophylaxis). TDF, FTC and EFV (Odimune, Tribuss, Atroiza and Atripla) as a single pill fixed dose combination (FDC) regimen are most commonly used to treat and prevent perinatal mother to child transmission (PMTCT) of HIV. AZT and NVP are the commonest drugs used for HIV prophylaxis during labour if patients received no ARVs antenatally. NVP syrup is given to infants postpartum and during breast feeding to prevent infection.

1-26 Which nucleoside and nucleotide reverse transcriptase inhibitors are commonly used?

Zidovudine (also called AZT) was the first ARV drug available. It is effective when used prophylactically during pregnancy and labour to reduce the risk of transmission of HIV from mother to infant. It can also be given to the newborn infant after delivery. When used alone for a short period it is uncommon for HIV to become resistant to AZT.

> NOTE AZT is a nucleoside analogue. This means that it mimics a natural nucleoside. Nucleosides are linked together to form DNA. When reverse transcriptase produces DNA, AZT is incorporated in preference to a natural nucleoside. The resulting DNA is not correctly formed and HIV cannot be produced.

AZT is well absorbed orally and crosses the placenta well. It increases the fetus's ability to resist infection from HIV. AZT needs to be taken twice a day.

3TC, TNF and FTC are commonly used and has the same mechanism of action as AZT. Common side effects of these drugs are shown in table 1-1.

1-27 Which non-nucleotide reverse transcriptase inhibitors are commonly used?

NVP is a potent and rapidly acting antiretroviral drug, which is very useful in reducing the risk of HIV transmission from mother to infant during labour and delivery. It is absorbed orally and crosses the placenta very well. A single dose is given to the mothers newly diagnosed to be HIV positive during labour or if ARV treatment has not yet been started. NVP has few adverse effects when used as a single dose. However, resistance develops rapidly when NVP is used as a single dose. Therefore, NVP always is used with Truvada (a combination of TDF and FTC) to prevent resistance developing.

. . . .

Prophylactic NVP is very useful in reducing the risk of mother-to-child transmission during labour and delivery for newly diagnosed mothers who are not yet on antiretroviral treatment.

. . . .

EFV is also a non-nucleoside reverse transcriptase inhibitor and commonly used together with TDF and FTC as a single FDC tablet taken once daily.

Table 1-1 Common side-effects of AZT, 3TC, FTC and TNF

AZT	3TC and FTC	TNF
• Headache • Malaise (feeling tired) • Muscle pains • Nausea and vomiting • Bone marrow suppression resulting in anaemia and neutropenia	• Headache • Nausea • Diarrhoea • Pancreatitis • Skin hyperpigmentation • Anaemia	• Vomiting and diarrhoea • Peripheral neuropathy • Osteoporosis • Lipodystrophy • Lactic acidosis • Renal failure

EFV is also used with AZT and 3TC as HAART when there are contra-indications to the use of TDF.

Common side effects of these drugs are shown in table 1-2.

1-28 Is a vaccine available to prevent HIV infection?

Unfortunately not. An effective vaccine against HIV is the only way that the HIV epidemic will be controlled. Many studies are being conducted in an attempt to produce an HIV vaccine. However it may be many years before an effective HIV vaccine is available.

1-29 What drugs are commonly used to prevent opportunistic infections?

1. Co-trimoxazole (Bactrim, Septran or Purbac) is currently used in patients with HIV infection to prevent opportunistic infections with Pneumocystis, Toxoplasma and some common bacteria. It is very effective but must be taken regularly. It is used with advanced disease when the CD4 count is 200 cells/μl or less and with stage 3 and 4 disease.
2. Isoniazid (INH) is used to prevent tuberculosis.

1-30 What is the general management of a patient with HIV infection?

The general management of adults with HIV infection consists of the following:

- A good, balanced diet to help prevent weight loss
- Prophylactic co-trimoxazole and INH when indicated
- Treat opportunistic infections if they occur.
- Monitor the clinical and immunological progress of the HIV infection.
- ARV drugs
- Emotional, social and financial support
- Manage the patient at a local primary-care clinic if possible.
- Prevent the spread of HIV to others.

Except for the use of ARV drugs, the general management of HIV infection is not expensive and makes a big difference to the quality of the patient's life. Whenever possible, the patient should not be admitted to hospital, but managed at home with the support of the community and primary healthcare services. Patients with AIDS should never be abandoned. AIDS cannot be effectively treated with diet alone.

Table 1-2 Common side-effects of NVP and EFV

NVP*	EFV
• Skin rash, that could be severe and life threatening (Stevens Johnson syndrome) • Hepatoxicity (liver damage) that could be severe and life threatening	• Dizzyness/drowsiness • Insomnia (unable to sleep) • Abnormal dreams • Psychiatric symptoms • Skin rash** • Hepatotoxicity** • Possible fetal harm during the 1st trimester

* Side effects do not occur if used as a single dose
* *Frequency of these side effects much lower compared with NVP

Accidental HIV infection

1-31 Are nurses and doctors at risk of infection when caring for HIV-positive women?

Yes, as body fluids, especially vaginal discharge and cervical secretions, blood, amniotic fluid, breast milk and semen may contain large amounts of HIV. Healthcare workers can become infected by HIV via the following routes:

- By needle-stick injuries or by cutting one's finger during surgery.
- Through sores or abrasions of the skin when handling body fluids.
- By splashes of body fluid into the eyes or mouth.
- Sweat, tears, saliva, sputum, vomitus, urine and stool is not infectious unless contaminated by above mentioned infectious body fluids.

1-32 How can healthcare workers reduce the risk of HIV infection?

By adopting standard (universal) precautions. This means that all body fluids should be regarded as potentially infectious in all patients. Precautions should always be taken to prevent exposure to infectious body fluids.

1-33 What are the standard precautions to prevent HIV infection when caring for patients?

All patients should be regarded as being potentially HIV positive. Therefore, general precautions should be taken with all patients. These precautions are especially important in patients known to be HIV positive.

- Wash your hands, or spray them with disinfectant, after touching a patient or after handling body fluids. Wash your hands with soap and water immediately should they become contaminated with blood.
- Use gloves when handling any body fluids, especially blood. Usually disposable, unsterile gloves can be used. Gloves do not have to be used when taking a blood sample.
- Wear a mask if there is a chance that body fluids may splash into your mouth.
- Wear protective glasses if there is a chance of blood splashing into your eyes. Be careful to avoid splashes.
- Wear a plastic apron or gown during procedures, such as a deliveries, when body fluid may soil your clothes. Remove the soiled apron or gown as soon as possible.
- Linen soiled with body fluids must be disposed of, usually into a special bag or container, until they can be sterilised. Gloves must be worn when handling soiled linen.
- All spilt blood must be cleaned up immediately and the surface wiped with a hypochlorite solution (Biocide, Milton or Jik mixed 2:1 with water). Use paper towels, which should then be placed in an approved disposal bag for incineration.
- All blood specimens for the laboratory must be placed in a leak-proof packet or container.
- Be very careful when handling 'sharps' (needles, blades, lancets).

Standard precautions should be adopted when managing all patients.

1-34 How should sharps be handled?

- Whenever sharps (needles, blades, lancets) are used, great care must be taken not to puncture or injure your skin.
- Handling of sharps should be reduced to a minimum.
- Needles must not be resheathed.
- Once used, always keep the sharp end of a needle, blade or lancet pointing away from you. Be careful not to stick anyone else.
- After withdrawing the sharp from the skin, immediately place it in a sharps container. The container must be within easy reach before starting the procedure. Failure to do this is the commonest way healthcare workers are infected with HIV while on duty.
- Never place a used sharp on the bed or work top.
- Correctly designed sharps containers must always be available. Do not allow them to become overfilled. They should be collected and be disposed of in a safe manner.
- When sutures are inserted always clamp the needle with the sharp tip against the needle holder when the needle is not being used.

Always use a sharps container for the disposal of lancets or needles.

1-35 What is the risk of HIV infection after an accidental needle-stick injury?

The overall risk without antiretroviral prophylaxis is 1 in 300. Therefore, of every 300 healthcare workers who prick or cut themselves with an instrument covered with HIV-positive blood, one person will become infected with HIV. With the correct use of antiretroviral prophylaxis this risk is reduced by 80%. The risk of infection is greatest if:

1. The wound is deep.
2. The person is stuck with a hollow needle.
3. The patient has AIDS or has recently been infected with HIV (high viral load).
4. Antiretroviral prophylaxis is not given or is given incorrectly.

The risk of infection without antiretroviral prophylaxis after a splash of HIV-infected blood into the mouth or eye, or contamination of a cut or skin abrasion, is less than 1 in 1000.

1-36 What prophylaxis should be given to a healthcare worker exposed accidentally to HIV?

Healthcare workers may be accidentally exposed to HIV by needle-stick injuries or splashes of infected body fluid into the eyes or mouth, or onto broken skin. The risk of infection is greatest with a cut or needle-stick injury. Every effort must be made to start antiretroviral prophylaxis within two hours of exposure. Start treatment as soon as possible. Treatment is probably not effective if the delay is greater than 72 hours.

Prophylaxis is strongly recommended with mucosal splashes if the patient is sick with AIDS. Prophylaxis is not indicated after exposure to uncontaminated, non-infectious body fluids.

One tablet of Truvada and one tablet of lopinavir/ritonavir (Aluvia) should be taken immediately and then continued for 28 days for prophylaxis. One tablet of Truvada contains TDF 300 mg and FTC 200 mg and is taken once daily. Aluvia contains lopinavir 400 mg and ritonavir 100mg and is taken 12-hourly. The adverse effects of nausea, vomiting, diarrhoea and tiredness are common. Therefore both drugs are best taken with food and an anti-emetic can be taken a half an hour before taking the tablets to reduce nausea.

Always acquaint yourself with the local post-exposure prophylaxis (PEP) protocol.

1-37 What is the correct procedure after a needle-stick injury?

After a needle-stick injury the following procedure should be followed:

1. Do not panic. Encourage bleeding from the puncture site and wash with soap and water. The mouth or eyes should immediately be washed with water after a blood splash.
2. Notify the correct hospital authority. Every hospital and clinic must have a clear management policy for accidental HIV exposure. This should be available to all staff. Everyone must know who the person to contact is, should accidental HIV exposure occur.
3. Start prophylactic antiretroviral management with Truvada and Aluvia as soon as possible. These drugs must be readily available in all hospitals and clinics both day and night.
4. Obtain consent and collect blood samples from the patient for HIV, and hepatitis C screening. If the health care worker has not been immunised also include a hepatitis B test. If consent is refused, assume that the patient is HIV positive. If the patient is under anaesthetic blood samples can be drawn, as provision is made for screening on consent forms for surgery. The patient must be informed when awake.
5. An HIV test need only be performed on the healthcare worker if the patient tests positive. A test for hepatitis B must always be done. This is to make sure that the healthcare worker is not already HIV positive and to test for immunity against hepatitis B. If the healthcare worker is HIV and hepatitis B positive, prophylaxis is not indicated.
6. Notify the laboratory that two urgent HIV tests are needed for screening. The screening test must be done as soon as possible. For medico legal purposed all screening must be laboratory tests and not rapid tests.
7. If the HIV test on the patient's blood is negative stop the antiretroviral prophylaxis. If the test is positive, continue for 28 days.
8. Liver function (ALT) and serum creatinine tests must be done at baseline and again at 2 and 6 weeks.

9. Repeat the HIV test on the healthcare worker after six weeks to determine whether or not he/she has become HIV positive. If the test is negative, repeat after another 3 and 6 months.

10. The efficacy of combined oral contraceptives is reduced by Aluvia. The health care worker must practice safe sex by using condoms until the HIV test at 6 months is negative.

11. Counselling and ongoing psychosocial support must be given for all healthcare workers exposed to HIV-contaminated blood.

All hospitals and clinics must keep emergency packs of prophylactic antiretrovirals for staff with accidental exposure to HIV.

Case study 1

During a public lecture at a social club, the speaker says that HIV infection in Africa is usually acquired by heterosexual intercourse. He also says that HIV infection is commoner in women. During question time a member of the public asks whether HIV is also spread by kissing. Another member of the audience asks if HIV infection is the same as having AIDS, and whether people who are HIV positive but well can be infectious to others.

1. Do you agree that HIV infection in Africa is usually acquired by heterosexual intercourse?

Yes. Heterosexual intercourse is the most common method of spreading HIV in Africa. However, the vertical spread from mother to infant is also very important. Homosexual intercourse and the use of contaminated needles are other important methods of spread in some communities.

2. Why is HIV infection commoner in women in Africa?

Because HIV is usually spread by unprotected heterosexual intercourse. As semen may remain in the vagina for some time after intercourse, women have a greater chance than men of being infected.

3. Can HIV be spread by kissing?

Probably not. HIV cannot be acquired by non-sexual contact such as social kissing, holding hands, hugging and sharing cooking and eating utensils.

4. Is HIV infection the same as having AIDS?

No. The difference commonly causes confusion among members of the public. Most people with HIV infection remain well for years before they become seriously sick with the illness called AIDS. Therefore, it is very common to have HIV infection without AIDS. With time, however, these people with asymptomatic HIV infection will become sick.

5. Can people who do not have AIDS transmit HIV to others?

Yes. Everyone with HIV infection is infectious to others even if they are clinically well. Patients on ARV treatment are less infectious than patients not receiving treatment.

Case study 2

A blood donor has a routine HIV test which is negative. A few weeks later she has unprotected sexual intercourse with a stranger she met in a night club. After three weeks she develops a fever, a mild cough and a generalised pink rash. On examination, her doctor notes that she has enlarged lymph nodes in her neck and axilla, and small ulcers on her throat. He diagnoses infectious mononucleosis and prescribes oral penicillin. She recovers rapidly. Six months later, when she again asks to donate blood, it is found that she is HIV positive.

1. What is the correct diagnosis of her illness?

Acute seroconversion illness. This occurs two to four weeks after HIV infection in about 50% of individuals. It is often misdiagnosed as acute infectious mononucleosis (glandular fever) as both conditions present with fever, sore throat, rash and lymphadenopathy.

2. How could she have avoided HIV infection?

By abstaining from sexual intercourse or by using a condom.

3. Can a person become infected with HIV by donating blood?

No. There is no risk in donating blood provided that a sterile needle is used. However, one can become infected by receiving blood donated by someone who is infected with HIV. Therefore, all donated blood in South Africa is screened for HIV.

4. For how long can this woman expect to remain well?

She will probably remain well for five to ten years. However, the latent phase of HIV infection may last as long as 15 years.

Case study 3

A young man presents with shortness of breath and a chronic cough. During the past few months he has noticed an unexplained weight loss. On examination he has oral thrush and generalised lymphadenopathy. A chest X-ray shows pneumonia with a cavity in one lung. The HIV rapid test is positive. Recently he was treated for syphilis.

1. What is the diagnosis?

Symptomatic HIV infection complicated by tuberculosis (TB). HIV infection commonly presents with a history of weight loss, cough and shortness of breath.

2. Is TB common in HIV-positive people?

Yes. It may be the first sign that the patient has symptomatic HIV disease.

3. Why has the patient got oral thrush?

Thrush is an infection caused by the fungus Candida. It is common in young infants but rare in adults. Thrush is one of the opportunistic infections which complicate HIV infection.

4. Why do patients with HIV disease commonly have opportunistic infections?

Because HIV damages the CD4 lymphocytes which play an important role in the immune system. Thrush, therefore, takes this opportunity of infecting the mouth. Some opportunistic infections, such as Pneumocystis and CMV, may also cause pneumonia which often presents with cough and shortness of breath.

5. How can syphilis increase the risk of becoming infected with HIV?

Often more than one sexually transmitted disease occurs in a patient. Syphilis causes genital ulcers that increase the risk of HIV infecting the person.

6. Can AIDS be treated?

AIDS can be treated with a combination of ARV drugs. While the signs and symptoms of AIDS may disappear while on treatment, HIV infection cannot be cured. A vaccine holds the only hope of ending the HIV epidemic.

Case study 4

After collecting capillary blood for glucose measurement from the heel of a newborn infant, a nurse accidentally pricks her finger with the lancet while cleaning up. A sharps container is not available in the nursery. She only informs the management the following day. Blood from the patient and the nurse is then sent urgently to the laboratory and the HIV test on the patient is positive. A one month course

of Truvada and Aluvia is started but she stops after a week as the medication makes her feel nauseous and tired.

1. What basic mistake was made by the nurse?

There was no sharps container in the nursery. After collecting a blood sample, the needle or lancet must immediately be placed in a special sharps container. It is extremely dangerous to place the used needle or lancet on the bed or work top, as staff commonly prick themselves while tidying up afterwards.

2. When should she have informed the management?

Immediately. As soon as any staff member pricks him- or herself with a blood-stained needle or lancet, the management must be informed so that the procedure of testing the patient's blood and starting prophylactic ARV drugs can begin without delay. Every hospital and clinic must have a clear list of instructions as to the correct procedure after a needle-stick injury.

3. Was the correct medication given?

Yes. A course of both Truvada and Aluvia are used for needle-stick injuries. However, the risk of HIV infection is increased if the treatment is not started within a few hours of the needle-stick injury.

4. What is the risk of her becoming infected with HIV?

Without treatment the risk is about 1 in 300. This risk is greatly reduced if the correct prophylactic treatment is started as soon as possible, preferably within two hours.

5. Does it matter that the prophylactic treatment was only taken for a week?

Yes. To be as effective as possible the treatment must be taken for 28 days.

Unfortunately the ARV agents do have adverse effects such as lethargy and nausea. As a result the full course of treatment is often not taken. Counseling regarding side effects of the drugs and measures to reduce side effects must always be given

2

HIV in pregnancy

Before you begin this unit, please take the corresponding test at the end of the book to assess your knowledge of the subject matter. You should redo the test after you've worked through the unit, to evaluate what you have learned.

Objectives

When you have completed this unit you should be able to:

- Assess the risk of HIV transmission from a woman to her fetus.
- Describe how pregnant women can be screened for HIV infection.
- List which pregnancy complications are commoner in women with HIV infection.
- Diagnose symptomatic HIV infection and AIDS in pregnancy.
- Use TDF, FTC and EFV as a single pill fixed dose (FDC) regimen to reduce the risk of vertical transmission.
- Manage a pregnant woman with HIV infection or AIDS.
- Understand the use of ARV treatment in pregnancy.

HIV infection in pregnancy

2-1 Is HIV infection common in pregnant women?

In Africa, where HIV infection is usually spread by sexual intercourse, HIV is more common in women than in men. In South Africa in the public health service during 1990 less than 1% of pregnant women were HIV positive. Then the prevalence increased rapidly, and has remained between 28 and 30% from 2004 onwards. The rates of infection vary widely from region to region. In some regions up to 40% of all pregnant women are HIV positive. Today about 260 000 HIV-positive women deliver infants in South Africa each year.

* *

Almost a third of pregnant women within the public health service in South Africa are HIV positive.

* *

2-2 Should pregnant women be screened for HIV?

Yes. All women should be tested for HIV when they first book for antenatal care. HIV infection in women is often diagnosed for the first time when they are screened during pregnancy. HIV screening is very important as it is the gateway to care. Therefore, women should book early for antenatal care and all should be offered screening for HIV infection. This should be done by 12 weeks of gestation or as soon as possible thereafter. In South Africa all pregnant women should be screened for HIV unless they ask not to be screened.

If the first HIV screen is negative, it should be repeated around 32 weeks gestation to detect any late infections.

....

All pregnant women should be offered HIV screening at 12 weeks gestation.

....

2-3 How may pregnant women be screened for HIV infection?

A blood test is used to screen for antibodies to HIV. The presence of HIV antibodies indicates the presence of HIV infection. A number of tests are available to screen for HIV antibodies. Usually the rapid test is used. Rapid tests are cheap, highly accurate and can be done on a drop of blood in the antenatal clinic. Two positive rapid tests, using kits from two different manufacturers on two separate blood samples, are needed before a definite diagnosis of HIV infection is made, in order to be sure that the diagnosis is correct.

2-4 Can HIV be transmitted from a pregnant woman to her fetus?

Yes. HIV can cross the placenta from mother to fetus at any time during pregnancy. Without antiretroviral (ARV) prophylaxis, the risk of

transmission up until the last few weeks of pregnancy is about 5%. However, most fetal infections during pregnancy takes places in late pregnancy or during labour and delivery. The combined risk of HIV transmission to the fetus during pregnancy, labour and delivery is about 20% if ARV prophylaxis is not used (5% during pregnancy and 15% during labour and vaginal delivery). The spread of HIV from a mother to her fetus or infant is called mother-to-child transmission (MTCT) or vertical transmission. Avoiding vertical transmission is one of the most important methods of preventing the spread of HIV in a community. In women who do not breastfeed, most vertical transmission takes place during labour and delivery.

NOTE HIV has been found as early as eight weeks of gestation in aborted fetuses. First trimester HIV infection may cause abortion and be more common than is presently believed. It is thought that the risk of HIV crossing the placenta in pregnancy increases in the last weeks of pregnancy as the lower segment is being formed.

2-5 Which HIV-positive women are at high risk of infecting their infants with HIV during pregnancy?

All HIV-positive women are at risk of infecting their fetus. However, the following women have the greatest risk of transmitting HIV to their fetus:

- Women who become infected with HIV during the pregnancy
- Women with clinical stage 3 or 4 HIV infection
- Women with a low CD4 count

- Women who are undernourished
- Women who do not have ARV prophylaxis

Women who become infected during pregnancy and women with advanced HIV infection have high viral loads that increase their risk of vertical transmission of HIV. It has been suggested that women who have an antepartum haemorrhage and women who have an amniocentesis may also have a higher risk of transmitting HIV to their infants.

2-6 What are the benefits of antenatal HIV screening?

1. The risk of HIV transmission to the fetus during pregnancy, labour and delivery can be reduced.
2. Women found to be HIV positive may decide to have a termination of pregnancy if before 13 weeks or with impaired health or extremely poor socio-economic circumstances if before 20 weeks gestation.
3. Women who are HIV negative can be reassured and be advised to practise safer sex to lower the risk of becoming infected.
4. Women who are HIV positive should be encouraged to practise safer sex to avoid infecting others.
5. Clinical signs of HIV infection may be detected early and complications treated in both the mother and her infant.
6. ARV prophylaxis or treatment with 3 drugs will be given to all HIV positive pregnant women.
7. Infants born to HIV-positive women can be correctly managed.

8. HIV-positive women can be counselled about infant feeding options while HIV-negative women should be encouraged to breastfeed.
9. HIV-positive women may decide not to have any more children.

All pregnant women should be counselled about the benefits of knowing their HIV status. This must be done at the first antenatal (booking) visit.

All pregnant women should be counselled about the benefits of knowing their HIV status.

2-7 Is consent needed for antenatal HIV screening?

Yes. Verbal consent must be obtained from all women before they are screened for HIV infection. Provider initiated counselling and testing will result in a high uptake of HIV testing. All antenatal women must be informed about investigations, specifically mentioning the HIV test that will routinely be done at the first antenatal visit. This information can be given in a group or individually. Thereafter each woman must be asked individually whether she wants a HIV test prior to taking blood. Women declining a HIV test must be referred to the counsellor for comprehensive counselling. This "opt out" method increases the number of women who are screened for HIV. Screening of individuals without their consent is a violation of human rights.

The results of the HIV screen must be added to the antenatal card so that, with shared confidentiality, all health workers caring for her and her infant know her status.

2-8 How should women be told the results of the screening test?

The results should be given privately to each woman. The implications of the results should be explained and post-test counselling offered if needed. Nurses, doctors, social workers or trained lay counsellors usually provide counselling. It is very important that breaking the news of a positive HIV status be done correctly. The rapid test gives the great benefit of same-day results which avoids a long wait for the test outcome.

2-9 When should termination of pregnancy be considered in HIV-positive women?

The option of termination of pregnancy should be discussed with HIV-positive women if the gestational age is less than 20 weeks. Most of these women will, however, elect to continue with their pregnancy, especially with ARV treatment now available.

The following should be taken into consideration when termination is discussed with the mother:

1. The stage of her HIV infection is important. Clinical signs of stage 3 or 4 infection indicate a much shorter life expectancy for the mother if adherence to ARV treatment is poor.

2. Other children and family members may have HIV infection and need care.
3. The family support structures. Who will look after this child if the mother becomes ill or dies?
4. The risk of the fetus or newborn infant becoming infected with HIV must be explained to the mother.

Every effort should be taken to prevent unplanned or unwanted pregnancies in HIV-positive women. The primary goal in preventing HIV infection is to prevent parents-to-be from becoming infected with HIV.

2-10 What precautions should HIV-negative women take to avoid becoming infected in pregnancy?

HIV-negative women should take precautions not to become infected with HIV both during pregnancy and breastfeeding. Becoming infected with HIV during pregnancy, or in the weeks before falling pregnant, places the fetus at high risk of also becoming infected. As with non-pregnant women, the best precaution is either not having sexual intercourse or to have intercourse with a single HIV-negative partner only. If both such sexual partners are faithful to each other and are not abusers of intravenous drugs, there is no risk of HIV infection. High-risk sexual activity by either partner, such as promiscuity, must be avoided at all costs during pregnancy and breastfeeding. If this is not possible then a condom must always be used.

2-11 Does HIV have an effect on the pregnancy?

Yes. Pregnancy complications are far commoner in women who are HIV positive. They occur most frequently in women with clinical signs of advanced HIV infection.

2-12 Which pregnancy complications are commoner in women who are HIV positive?

1. Infections
   - Pulmonary and extra-pulmonary tuberculosis
   - Other sexually transmitted diseases
   - Urinary tract infection
   - Pneumonia
   - Opportunistic infections
   - Severe chicken pox or shingles (Varicella zoster infections)

NOTE Any pregnant woman who presents with pneumonia must be suspected of having HIV infection.

2. Early pregnancy complications
   - Abortion (miscarriage)
   - Ectopic pregnancy
3. Late pregnancy complications
   - The risk of stillbirth is doubled
   - Chorioamnionitis
   - Intra-uterine growth restriction, especially if the mother is underweight
   - Abruptio placentae
   - Anaemia
   - Preterm labour and prelabour rupture of the membranes, especially if chorioamnionitis is present

NOTE As a result of pregnancy complications, the neonatal mortality rate is increased fivefold if the mother has advanced HIV infection (AIDS).

2-13 Are there any procedures in pregnancy which may increase the risk of HIV transmission?

Amniocentesis and external cephalic version may possibly increase the risk of vertical transmission. Amniocentesis should only be done if there is a good indication and there is easy access to a pool of amniotic fluid, without having to pass through the placenta. ARV prophylaxis with 3 drugs should be started 2 weeks, but preferably 4 weeks before the procedure if the woman is not already on ARV prophylaxis or treatment. Both procedures will be safe if women are on ARV prophylaxis and known to have non-detectable viral loads.

HIV prophylaxis and treatment in pregnancy

2-14 What is the benefit of antiretroviral drugs in pregnancy?

ARV drugs can be used in two different ways during pregnancy:

1. ARV drugs can be used *prophylactically* to reduce the risk of HIV transmission from mother to infant during pregnancy, labour and breast feeding, i.e. prevention of mother-to-child transmission (PMTCT).
2. ARV *treatment* (therapy) to both treat HIV infection in the mother and reduce the risk of HIV transmission to her infant.

2-15 How effective is antiretroviral prophylaxis in reducing HIV transmission?

The use of prophylactic ARV drugs during pregnancy, labour and delivery reduces the risk of HIV transmission from mother to infant. If ARV prophylaxis is given, the transmission rate during pregnancy, labour and delivery for non-breastfeeding women can be reduced from 20% to less than 2%. The risk of transmission is lowest if 3 ARV drugs are used for women with CD4 counts of 350 cells/ml or less. The risk of transmission through breastfeeding if on 3 ARV drugs is about 0,2% per month of breastfeeding.

HIV transmission during pregnancy, labour and delivery is less than 2% when prophylaxis with 3 antiretroviral drugs is used.

2-16 Which antiretroviral drugs are used prophylactically in pregnancy?

The most commonly used drug to reduce the risk of mother-to-infant transmission during pregnancy is TDF (tenofovir) FTC (emtricitabine) and EFV (efavirenz) as a single pill fixed dose (FDC) regimen.

TDF, FTC and EFV as a single fixed dose combination (FDC) regimen are the ARV drugs of choice for HIV prophylaxis and treatment during pregnancy.

NOTE Trade names of the fixed dose pill of TDF, FTC and EFV include Odimune, Tribuss, Atoiza and Atripla

2-17 How can antiretroviral drugs be used in pregnancy to reduce the risk of vertical transmission of HIV?

ARV drugs can be used a number of ways to reduce the risk of mother-to-child transmission of HIV.

1. **Prophylactic** ARV with 3 drugs as a single pill fixed dose (FDC) regimen is started at 14 weeks of pregnancy when women are diagnosed to be HIV positive and are healthy with a CD4 count above 350 cells/ml and no signs of stage 3 or 4 disease. Once the risk of transmission of HIV no longer exists, i.e. the mother has weaned her infant or decided to formula feed, the ARV drugs for prophylaxis are stopped. This management is according to the World Health Organisation (WHO) Option B programme. The use of prophylactic ARV drugs aims at preventing HIV transmission rather than treating the mother.

2. **Treatment** (therapy) with ARV drugs is given to both treat HIV infection in the woman and reduce the risk of HIV transmission to her infant. ARV treatment with 3 drugs as a single pill fixed dose (FDC) regimen is started when pregnant women are diagnosed to be HIV positive with a CD4 count below 350 cells/ml or with signs of stage 3 or 4 disease. Unlike ARV prophylaxis, ARV treatment is continued for life

3. A third option is that ARV treatment may also be started in **all HIV positive women** irrespective of their CD4 count and the stage of the disease. Again the treatment is continued for life. This management of all HIV positive pregnant women is according to the WHO Option B+ programme.
4. The use of AZT during pregnancy, and AZT followed by a single dose NVP during labour, is according to the WHO Option A programme. This regimen is used when pregnant women decline taking 3 ARV drugs, defaulted their treatment or are only diagnosed to be HIV positive during labour. After delivery these women should be started on Option B or B+.
5. All above regimen reduces the risk of HIV transmission by reducing the viral load in the maternal blood.

NOTE: Some countries have implemented WHO Option B and some B+. In South Africa 8 provinces have implemented Option B and the Western Cape Province Option B+.

It is best to start prophylactic FDC at 14 weeks gestation if women are healthy and do not require ARV drugs for their own health.

2-18 What is the dose of FDC?

FDC a single pill fixed dose regimen that consist of TDF 300 mg, FTC 200mg and EFV 600 mg. One FDC pill is taken once a day at bedtime (and not at suppertime).

2-19 What is the dose of AZT when used for prophylaxis during pregnancy?

If AZT is used alone to reduce the risk of HIV transmission during pregnancy (WHO Option A) the dose is 300 mg (three 100 mg capsules twice a day).

2-20 Can EFV cause congenital abnormalities or harm the fetus?

There is a concern about a possible association between use of EFV in the first trimester of pregnancy and congenital abnormalities. If HIV is diagnosed early in pregnancy, the recommendation is to start FDC only at 14 weeks if the mother is healthy and does not require ARV drugs for her own health. If the woman is already taking EFV when she falls pregnant she should continue with the same treatment.

2-21 What is the role of vitamins in reducing vertical transmission of HIV?

There is no evidence that giving vitamins, especially vitamin A, during pregnancy reduces the risk of vertical transmission of HIV from mother to fetus in most communities. A high dose of vitamin A during the first trimester may cause congenital abnormalities. Therefore, if women take vitamins during pregnancy, they should not take more than one multivitamin tablet a day.

HIV and AIDS during pregnancy

2-22 Is AIDS an important cause of maternal death?

As the HIV epidemic spreads, the number of pregnant women dying of advanced HIV infection (AIDS) has increased dramatically. In some countries, such as South Africa, AIDS is now the commonest cause of maternal death.

NOTE The Third and Fourth Triennial Report on Confidential Enquiries into Maternal Deaths in South Africa (2005 to 2010) showed that AIDS was the commonest cause of maternal death. Many additional AIDS deaths may have been missed, when HIV testing was not done.

AIDS is the commonest cause of maternal death in South Africa.

2-23 Does pregnancy increase the risk of progression from asymptomatic to symptomatic HIV infection and AIDS?

Pregnancy appears to have little or no effect on the progression from asymptomatic to symptomatic HIV infection. However, in women who already have symptomatic HIV infection, pregnancy may lead to a more rapid progression from stage 3 to 4 disease.

Progression of HIV infection during pregnancy can be monitored by:

1. Laboratory tests
2. Clinical signs

2-24 Which laboratory tests indicate the progression of HIV infection?

1. A falling CD4 count is an important marker of progression in HIV. It is an indicator of the degree of damage to the immune system. The normal CD4 count is 700 to 1100 cells/µl. A CD4 count below 200 cells/µl indicates severe damage to the immune system.
2. A high viral load indicates a large number of virus particles in the blood and gives an idea as to how fast the HIV infection is progressing to AIDS. This test is used to monitor the response to treatment.

The CD4 count is an important marker of HIV progression during pregnancy.

2-25 How is the clinical severity of HIV infection classified?

The World Health Organisation (WHO) classification of clinical staging is used in both pregnant and non-pregnant individuals. Stage 1 is very mild while stage 4 is most severe. Life expectancy is best with stage 1 and worst with stage 4.

WHO staging is as follows:

Stage 1: Clinically well. Generalised lymphadenopathy may be present.

Stage 2: Mild weight loss or minor rashes or recurrent upper respiratory tract infections.

Stage 3: Moderate weight loss with oral thrush, pulmonary tuberculosis (TB), or severe bacterial infections.

Stage 4: Severe HIV-associated (opportunistic) infections (i.e. atypical pneumonia, esophageal thrush, extrapulmonary TB) cancer and wasting.

HIV infection is classified clinically into four stages.

Stage 4 HIV disease is also called AIDS. Therefore the complications seen in stage 4 are called 'AIDS-defining conditions'. This is confusing to many as the word 'AIDS' is often used incorrectly to mean any stage of HIV infection where a women have symptoms and signs of illness.

Women with stage 4 HIV infection have AIDS.

2-26 Can an HIV-positive woman be cared for in a primary-care clinic?

Most women who are HIV positive are clinically well with a normal pregnancy. Others may only have minor problems (grade 1 or 2). These women can usually be cared for in a primary-care clinic throughout their pregnancy, labour and puerperium provided their pregnancy is normal and their CD4 count is 350 cells/μl or more. Women with pregnancy complications should be referred to hospital as would be done with HIV-negative women. Women with HIV-related problems who do not respond to treatment at a primary-care clinic may have to be referred to an HIV/ARV (antiretroviral) clinic where staff are trained to care for women with

more severe HIV infection. Due to the large numbers of women, the HIV/ARV clinics cannot see all pregnant women who have minor problems related to HIV infection.

Most HIV-positive women who are clinically well during their pregnancy with a CD4 count of 350 or more can usually be cared for at a primary-care clinic.

It is very important that the primary-care clinic and the HIV clinic work in close partnership. Maternal and HIV care must be integrated.

The primary-care clinic and the HIV clinic must work together in a close partnership.

2-27 How are pregnant women with HIV infection managed at a primary-care clinic?

In a country with limited healthcare resources the management of women with HIV infection or AIDS in pregnancy is restricted to affordable protocols. The management of pregnant women is different to that of non-pregnant adults. All women with CD4 counts of 350 cell/ml and less or stage 3 of 4 disease should be started on treatment with 3 ARV drugs for life. The most important step is to identify those pregnant women who are HIV positive.

The principles of management of pregnant women with HIV infection at a primary-care clinic are:

1. Make the diagnosis of HIV infection by offering routine HIV screening to all pregnant women at the start of their antenatal care.
2. Assess the CD4 count in all HIV-positive women as soon as their HIV status is known.
3. Screen for tuberculosis and clinical signs of HIV infection at each antenatal visit.
4. A cervical cytology (PAP) smear should be done if the woman has not had a smear reported to be normal within the last year. If the woman is already 32 weeks or more pregnant the smear needs to be postponed to the 6 weeks postnatal visit.
5. Good diet. Nutritional support may be needed.
6. Emotional support and counselling.
7. Prevention of mother-to-child transmission (PMTCT) of HIV.
8. Start all women on 3 ARV drugs using FDC.
9. Treating HIV with 3 ARV drugs is also called Highly Active Antiretroviral Treatment or HAART.

All HIV-positive women should have their CD4 count measured.

2-28 Which health workers should care for women with HIV infection?

Most women with HIV infection can be cared for by nurses at a primary-care clinic. Even in hospital, much of the care can be done by nurses. Nurse-initiated ARV treatment is essential if the large numbers of pregnant women needing treatment are to be adequately managed. Doctors should support the nurses and help with complicated problems.

Clinical staging of HIV infection

2-29 What clinical signs suggest stage 1 and 2 HIV infection?

1. Women with stage 1 disease are generally well but may have persistent generalised lymphadenopathy.
2. Women with stage 2 disease may have:
   • Repeated or chronic mouth or genital ulcers
   • Extensive skin rashes
   • Repeated upper respiratory tract infections such as otitis media or sinusitis
   • Herpes zoster (shingles)

Most of these women can be managed at a primary-care clinic. These clinical problems are usually treated symptomatically with simple drugs which are not expensive.

2-30 What are the important features suggesting stage 3 HIV infection?

Features of stage 3 HIV infection include:

1. Unexplained weight loss. Pregnant women normally gain rather than lose weight.
2. Oral candidiasis (thrush)
3. Cough, fever and night sweats suggesting pulmonary tuberculosis
4. Cough, fever and shortness of breath suggesting bacterial pneumonia
5. Chronic diarrhoea or unexplained fever for more than one month
6. Severe or repeated bacterial infections, especially pneumonia

It is important to think of these HIV-associated conditions at every clinic visit. These women may need to be referred to an HIV clinic for further investigation and management. Pulmonary tuberculosis is common in women with HIV infection. Women with pulmonary tuberculosis have stage 3 disease irrespective of their clinical condition or CD4 count.

Pulmonary tuberculosis is common in women with symptomatic HIV infection.

2-31 What are the important features suggesting stage 4 HIV infection?

Features of stage 4 HIV infection include:

1. Severe weight loss
2. AIDS-defining illnesses such as:
   - Severe HIV-associated (opportunistic) infections
   - Malignancies such as Kaposi's sarcoma

Common, severe opportunistic infections include:

- Oesophageal candidiasis which presents with difficulty swallowing
- Pneumocystis pneumonia which presents with cough, fever and shortness of breath
- Cryptococcal meningitis and toxoplasmosis of the brain (encephalitis) present with headache, vomiting and confusion
- Extrapulmonary tuberculosis (TB)

It is important to recognise the signs of stage 3 and 4 HIV infection.

2-32 What are the principles of managing pregnant women with AIDS?

In addition to the steps in the management of all HIV-positive women, the following should be done at the HIV/ARV clinic:

Prophylactic co-trimoxazole (one tablet per day) to prevent Pneumocystis pneumonia and some bacterial infections. Prophylactic co-trimoxazole 2 tablets daily are given when the CD4 count is less than 200 cells/ml to prevent peumocystis pneumonia. Women with any of these signs of stage 4 HIV infection must be urgently referred to hospital.

1. Treatment of opportunistic and other bacterial infections, such as pneumonia and urinary tract infections
2. Multivitamin supplements
3. If active tuberculosis is diagnosed, treatment must be started
4. Urgently prepare the woman for ARV treatment
5. Start ARV treatment according to the correct protocol
6. Monitor the progress on ARV treatment

NOTE TB prophylaxis with INH is often provided.

Use of antiretroviral (ARV) treatment in pregnancy

2-33 What is antiretroviral treatment?

Lifelong ARV treatment is the use of three or more ARV drugs in combination to treat women with severe HIV infection or AIDS. The aim of ARV treatment is to lower the viral load and allow the immune system to recover. ARV treatment is rolled out to all South Africans who need it. This require extensive strengthening of the primary-care system in South Africa.

2-34 What are the indications for antiretroviral treatment in pregnancy?

All pregnant women who are HIV positive need to be commenced on a single pill fixed dose (FDC) regimen. If managed according the Option B+ programme, women will remain on ARV treatment for life. If managed according the Option B programme FDC is stopped following weaning or postpartum for formula feeding mothers. Mothers managed according to Option B, however, remain on ARV treatment if any of the following should develop:

1. Clinical signs of stage 3 or 4 HIV infection
2. A CD4 count of 350 cells/µl or below
3. Tuberculosis

Pregnant women who progress to stage 3 or 4 HIV infection or a CD count of 350 cells/µl or below while on option B during pregnancy should remain on ARV treatment for life.

2-35 What preparation is needed for antiretroviral treatment?

Preparing a woman to start ARV treatment is very important. This requires education, counselling and social assessment before ARV treatment can be started. These women need to learn about their illness and the importance of excellent adherence (taking their ARV drugs at the correct time every day) and regular clinic attendance. They also need to know the side effects of ARV drugs and how to recognise them. Careful general examination and some blood tests are also needed before starting ARV treatment. If there is doubt about readiness of women to commence ARV treatment, they could be asked to come back after a day or two for further counseling and to then start treatment.

2-36 What drugs are used for antiretroviral treatment during pregnancy?

Usually ARV treatment is provided to pregnant women in South Africa with a single pill fixed dose (FDC) regimen consisting of three drugs:

- TDF
- FTC
- EFV

This is the national first-line standard drug combination used during pregnancy. Women already on a different ARV regimen should:

- Switch to FDC if on TDF/ lamuvidine (3TC)/EFV
- Remain on their current regimen if on AZT/3TC/EFV, stavudine (d4T)/3TC/EFV or TDF/3TC/ nevirapine (NVP)

Women who do not respond to first-line treatment, or have severe side effects to the drugs used in first-line treatment, may have to be considered for second-line treatment with either AZT, 3TC and lopinavir/ritonavir (LPV/r) or Truvada and lopinavir/ ritonavir (LPV/r). Truvada is a combination of TDF 300 mg and FTC 200 mg as a single tablet taken once daily. LPV/r is taken as two tablets 12 hourly.

NOTE LPV/r is a combination of 200 mg LPV and 50 mg ritonavir in a single tablet.

2-37 Is it dangerous for a woman to fall pregnant if she is already receiving antiretroviral treatment?

No. If a woman is already on ARV treatment when she falls pregnant:

Women who fall pregnant while receiving standard first-line therapy with a single pill fixed dose (FDC) regimen may continue the medication throughout pregnancy.

Women receiving standard second-line therapy should also continue the medication throughout pregnancy. Most women who are clinically well on ARV treatment when they fall pregnant

remain well with few treatment problems during their pregnancy. Women already on a different ARV regimen should:

- Switch to FDC if on TDF/ lamuvidine (3TC)/EFV
- Remain on their current regimen if on AZT/3TC/EFV, stavudine (d4T)/3TC/EFV or TDF/3TC/ nevirapine (NVP)

2-38 When can pregnant women be started on antireroviral treatment?

ARV treatment should be started on the day of diagnosis. If HIV is diagnosed early in pregnancy, the recommendation is to commence FDC only at 14 weeks if the mother is healthy and does not require ARV drugs for her own health. However, it is best to start treatment as soon as possible, in women who are seriously ill or with a CD4 count less than 50 cells/μl.

2-39 Can antiretroviral treatment be started close to term?

Yes, the FDC regimen could be started close to term. This would be especially important for women seriously ill or with a CD4 count is less than 50 cells/μl.

Healthy women who present close to term may be given prophylaxis with AZT 300 mg 12 hourly during the remaining few days or week of pregnancy and AZT 300mg 3 hourly and single dose NVP 200mg during labour according to Option A. A single tablet of Truvada is taken together with the single dose NVP in labour to prevent resistance developing against NVP. The mother will then be started on FDC following the delivery.

NOTE The viral load starts reducing following 2 weeks of FDC and will mostly be low following 4 weeks of treatment.

2-40 What are the benefits of antiretroviral treatment during pregnancy?

1. ARV treatment improves the health of the mother and prevents her dying from HIV infection during or soon after pregnancy.
2. ARV treatment also reduces the risk of vertical transmission.
3. Women on ARV treatment can be kept alive and well for many years, enabling them to care for their children and be economically active. Therefore the number of AIDS orphans will be significantly reduced.

2-41 What are the side effects of antiretroviral treatment?

Pregnant women on ARV treatment may have side effects to the drugs. These are usually mild and occur during the first six weeks of treatment. However, side effects may occur at any time that women are on ARV treatment. It is important that the staff at primary-care clinics are aware of these side effects and that they ask for symptoms and look for signs at each clinic visit. Side effects are more common with ARV treatment than with ARV prophylaxis during pregnancy.

Common early side effects during the first few weeks of starting ARV prophylaxis or treatment include:

1. Lethargy, tiredness and headaches
2. Nausea, vomiting and diarrhoea
3. Muscle pains and weakness

More severe side effects of some ARV drugs, which can be fatal, include renal impairment, lactic acidosis, hepatitis, anaemia and pancreatitis.

Drugs specific side effects are:

- TDF can cause renal impairment or even renal failure. Lactic acidosis is a rare but serious side effect of TDF. It presents with weight loss, tiredness, nausea, vomiting, abdominal pain and shortness of breath in women who have been well on ARV treatment for a few months
- Other she side effects of TDF are vomiting and diarrhea, peripheral neuropathy, osteoporosis, lipodystrophy and, lactic acidosis.
- EFV may cause drowsiness, dizziness, abnormal dreams, psychiatric symptoms, skin rash and hepatotoxicity. EFV may make active psychiatric disease worse.
- The side effects of FTC are headache, nausea, diarrhea, pancreatitis, skin hyperpigmentation and anaemia.
- The side effects of AZT are headache, malaise (feeling tired), muscle pains, nausea, vomiting and bone marrow suppression resulting in anaemia and neutropenia.
- Nevirapine may cause severe skin rashes and hepatitis. With severe skin rashes, especially with blisters, the NVP must be stopped and the woman must be referred urgently to the HIV/ARV clinic. Hepatitis can be

caused by all ARV drugs but especially nevirapine.

Staff at primary-care clinics must be aware and look out for these very important side effects. Like most drugs, FDC has side effects. These are a combination of the side effects of each of the 3 drugs. FDC should be taken at bedtime in the evening with a glass of water. In this way the drowsiness and dizziness caused by EFV will be avoided.

NOTE Stavudine (d4T) was part of first line ARV treatment in the past and commonly caused side effect, including lactic acidosis.

. . . .
Antiretroviral treatment can have severe side effects
. . . .

2-42 What are contra-indications to the use of antiretroviral drugs?

TDF is contraindicated in chronic renal disease as it can cause renal failure if renal impairment is already present. TDF is also contraindicated if there is a history of chronic hypertension, diabetes, previous hospitalization for kidney disease or if one plus or more proteinuria is present on urine dipstix.

NOTE With a history of possible chronic renal disease, a serum creatinine concentration should be requested and the woman started on AZT prophylaxis. If the serum creatinine is 85 µmol/l or more shet must remain on AZT if the CD4 count is above 350 cells/ml andbe managed according to Option A, or she should be started on an AZT, 3TC and EFV regimen if the CD4 count is 350 cells/ml or less. If the serum creatinine

is less than 85 µmol/l a TDF containing regimen could be used, with careful follow-up of the serum creatinine.

EFV is contra-indicated in any women with active psychiatric illness. Mild depression is not a contra-indication for the use of EFV.

NOTE With active psychiatric illness give AZT according to Option A if the CD4 count is above 350 cells/ml or commenced Truvada and NVP or AZT, 3TC and NVP if the CD4 count is 350 cells/ml or less

As AZT can cause anaemia, a laboratory hemoglobin concentration should be done at the start of treatment. Women with a haemoglobin concentration below 8 g/dl should not be given AZT.

. . . .
TDF should not be used if there is renal disease, EFV with psychiatric illness or AZT with severe anaemia.
. . . .

2-43 What blood tests should be done to monitor antiretroviral treatment during pregnancy?

1. The serum creatinine value must be measured before starting an ARV regimen containing TDF. This drug should not be used if the serum creatinine is 85 µmol/l or more or a creatinine clearance of 50 ml/l or less. The serum creatinine is repeated at 3 months, 6 and 12 months following initiation of treatment.
2. As AZT can cause anaemia, these women should have a full blood count at the start of treatment and

then a laboratory haemoglobin measurement done every month for 3 months and then 3 monthly during the rest of pregnancy. Women with a haemoglobin concentration below 8 g/dl should not be given AZT.

3. An ARV regimen containing NVP requires a serum ALT (alanine aminotransferase liver function test) to be done at the start of treatment (baseline) and again at two and four weeks. Thereafter ALT should be measured monthly until delivery.

2-44 Who should follow up on women on antiretroviral treatment during pregnancy?

Whenever possible, a pregnant woman on ARV treatment should be followed up at the clinic or hospital where she is receiving antenatal care. Only women with serious problems related to their HIV infection or ARV treatment need be referred to a special HIV clinic.

At every visit these women must be encouraged and supported to continue with excellent drug adherence. They should also be monitored for clinical signs of HIV infection and side effects of ARV treatment, as well as having their serum creatinine (if in TDF) and haemoglobin (if on AZT) monitored.

TB/HIV co-infection

2-45 How is TB/HIV co-infection diagnosed?

All pregnant women, especially if they have HIV infection, should be asked about the symptoms of tuberculosis at every antenatal visit. These are:

- Cough of any duration
- Fever
- Severe night sweats
- Weight loss

2-46 How is the diagnosis of pulmonary tuberculosis confirmed?

Three sputum specimens should be sent for microscopy and culture. A single posterior anterior chest x-ray is requested with the fetus screened off with a lead apron. If enlarged lymph nodes are palpable a fine needle aspiration should be requested for microscopy and a culture.

NOTE GeneXpert testing for tuberculosis has replaced conventional cultures and results are available within one day.

2-47 When should anti-TB treatment be started?

Pulmonary tuberculosis is a feature of stage 3 disease in women with HIV infection. Therefore they need both anti-TB treatment and be started on lifelong ARV treatment:

First start anti-TB treatment for two weeks and only then begin ARV treatment. FDC will usually be used for treatment but prophylaxis with AZT is given during the 2 weeks when FDC is not given.

If women develop tuberculosis while on lifelong ARV treatment, anti-TB treatment can be started without delay.

The risk of side effects is increased when ARV and anti-TB drugs are used together, especially if the tuberculosis has been treated for less than two weeks when the ARV drugs are started.

NOTE Commencing anti-TB treatment and ARV treatment together increases the risk of TB associated immune reconstitution inflammatory syndrome (TB IRIS).

2-48 How is a woman with tuberculosis treated in pregnancy?

If possible, antenatal care, HIV management and anti-TB treatment should be integrated at a primary-care clinic. Treatment is usually started with rifampicin, INH, pyrizinamide and ethambutol. These 4 drugs are combined in Rifafour and taken as 4 tablets per day.

The dose of LPV/r should be doubled if receiving both anti-TB treatment and an ARV regimen containing LPV/r as rifampicin lowers the blood levels of both LPV/r and NVP. Therefore, NVP is replaced by EFV if an ARV regimen containing NVP is used.

Case study 1

A woman with an unplanned pregnancy books for antenatal care at 8 weeks of gestation. During screening she is found to be HIV positive. She is clinically well. After counseling, blood for a CD4 count is taken. She is then started immediately on FDC and asked to come back for a follow-up visit in 4 weeks time.

1. What should have been discussed with her in addition to post test counselling following a positive HIV test?

The possibility of termination of her pregnancy should been discussed. She is less than 13 weeks pregnant and the pregnancy is unplanned.

2. Should FDC have been started at the first visit?

No, she is healthy and early in the 1st trimester of her pregnancy. Starting FDC could have been delayed until 14 weeks. FDC contains EFV and there are concerns about the safety of EFV in the 1st trimester of pregnancy.

3. Which additional special investigations should have been requested at the first antenatal visit because she is to start on ARV treatment with FDC?

In addition to the routine blood tests done at the first antenatal visit a serum creatinine concentration should have been requested. FDC contains TDF that could cause renal impairment and is contraindicated with women that have chronic renal disease.

4. When would the serum creatinine concentration will be a contraindication to the use of TDF?

A serum creatinine concentration of 85 μmol/l or more.

5. Was a follow-up date in 4 weeks time, the correct management?

No, HIV positive women are always asked to come again in one week's time for follow-up of the CD4 count. Healthy women may have an unexpected low CD4 count that would require FDC to be started without delay.

Case study 2

A woman who is clinically well is found to be HIV positive when screened during her first antenatal visit at 20 weeks gestation. She is started on ARV prophylaxis with AZT and asked to come back in one week's time. When she is seen one week later her CD4 count is 400 cells/μl. She is reassured that she has stage 1 disease and a CD4 count above the threshold to start ARV treatment and therefore should continue with AZT only.

1. Is she correctly managed according the new WHO guidelines?

No, she should have been started on FDC, a single pill fixed dose regimen containing 3 ARV drugs (TDF, FTC and EFV) according the WHO Option B or B+ regimens.

2. What contraindications are there to the use of FDC?

TDF is contraindicated in chronic renal disease as it can cause renal failure if renal impairment is already present. TDF is also contraindicated if there is a history of chronic hypertension, diabetes, previous hospitalization for kidney disease or if there is one plus or more proteinuria on urine dipstix. EFV is contra-indicated with psychiatric illness and any women with active psychiatric disease should not receive EFV. Mild depression is not a contraindication for the use of EFV.

3. What contraindications are there to the use of AZT?

AZT can cause anaemia. Therefore women with a haemoglobin concentration below 8 g/dl should not be given AZT.

4. Which special investigates are required if a women is taking AZT as prophylaxis or placed on an ARV regimen containing AZT?

A laboratory hemoglobin concentration should be done at the start of treatment and every month during pregnancy for 3 months and then 3 monthly.

5. During a follow-up visit after two months she is asymptomatic and clinically well but has enlarged lymph nodes palpable in her neck, axillas and groins. She is reassured that this is no reason for concern and that routine follow-up could continue. Is this management correct?

The information provided to the woman is correct. With stage 1 disease women are clinically well but a generalised lymphadenopathy may be present.

Case study 3

When booking for antenatal care at 24 weeks gestation, a woman who is clinically well is found to be HIV positive on routine screening. She is started on ARV treatment with FDC and asked to come back in one week's time. When she is seen one week later she complains of nausea and has had diarrhoea a few times daily. She also feels lethargic. Her CD4 count is 300 cells/µl. She is advised to stop her FDC temporarily until the side effects of the drugs have stopped.

1. Are these side effects to be expected when starting on FDC?

Yes, common early side effects during the first few weeks of starting ARV treatment include: lethargy, tiredness and headaches, nausea, vomiting and diarrhea, muscle pains and weakness.

2. Should ARV treatment be stopped if these side effects occur?

These are mild side effects and usually disappear on their own. They can be treated symptomatically. It is important that ARV treatment is continued even if there are mild side effects.

3. During counselling regarding infant feeding options later during the pregnancy, the woman indicates that she would like to breastfeed her infant. She is told that she needs to continue with the FDC until one week following weaning. As she is clinically well should she then stop the FDC?

The woman should not stop the FDC. According to the Option B programme, only women that do not require ARV drugs for their own health should stop FDC following weaning. As she has a CD4 count less than 350 cells/ml she must remain on FDC for life.

4. Why is it important that she continues with FDC for life?

A CD4 count 350 cells/ml or less indicates some degree of immunologic impairment has already occurred. Without ARV treatment she is at risk of progressing to stage 3 or 4 disease in the near future. Keeping the mother healthy is of great importance as the health of the infant also depends on a healthy mother.

Case study 4

A woman is found to be HIV positive when screened during her first antenatal visit at 22 weeks gestation. She complains of a cough, feeling feverish at times and that she has heavy night sweats. These symptoms have been present for a few weeks. As she is clearly not healthy, she is started on FDC without delay.

1. What co-infection should be considered with this womant?

She has a cough, fever and night sweats. The presence of any one of these symptoms requires tuberculosis to be excluded before starting FDC.

2. Which measures should have been taken to exclude tuberculosis prior to commencing FDC?

Three sputum specimens should be sent for microscopy and culture. A single posterior anterior chest x-ray is requested with the fetus screened off with a lead apron. If enlarged lymph nodes are palpable a fine needle aspiration should be requested for microscopy and a culture.

3. If she is diagnoses with tuberculosis, could she be started on anti-TB treatment and FDC at the same time?

Anti-TB treatment must be given for two weeks and then FDC could be started. Prophylaxis with AZT is given during those 2 weeks. The risk of side effects is increased whenARV and anti-TB drugs are used together, especially if the tuberculosis has been treated for less than two weeks when the ARV drugs are started.

4. Could anti-TB drugs and FDC be taken together?

Yes, the anti-TB drugs do not influence the blood levels of TDF, FTC and EFV which make up FDC. Anti-TB drugs do lower the blood levels of LPV/r and NVP.

3

HIV during labour and delivery

Before you begin this unit, please take the corresponding test at the end of the book to assess your knowledge of the subject matter. You should redo the test after you've worked through the unit, to evaluate what you have learned.

Objectives

When you have completed this unit you should be able to:

• Explain the risk of HIV transmission to the infant during labour and delivery.
• Identify women at the greatest risk of transmitting HIV to their infant.
• List ways of reducing the risk of HIV transmission to the infant.
• Describe how to use antiretroviral drugs during labour.
• Reduce the risk of HIV infection of the staff during labour and delivery.
• Provide family planning advice to HIV-positive women after delivery.

HIV transmission during labour

3-1 Can HIV be transmitted from mother to infant during labour and delivery?

Yes. During labour and delivery the infant is exposed to cervical and

vaginal secretions as well as maternal blood, all of which may contain HIV that can infect the infant. Without ARV prophylaxis or treatment, there is a risk of HIV transmission from a mother to her fetus is during labour and vaginal delivery.

3-2 What is the risk of an infant being infected with HIV during labour and delivery without antiretroviral prophylaxis or treatment?

The risk of HIV transmission from mother to infant during pregnancy, labour and vaginal delivery together is about 20% if ARV prophylaxis or treatment is not used. The risk of HIV transmission during labour and vaginal delivery alone is about 15%. Therefore, most of this transmission takes place during labour and delivery. Therefore efforts to reduce HIV transmission during labour and delivery are very important.

• •
Most vertical spread of HIV takes place during labour and vaginal delivery if antiretroviral prophylaxis or treatment is not used.
• •

3-3 Can HIV infection be diagnosed for the first time during labour?

If a woman has not been screened for HIV during her pregnancy, she can still be screened during labour using a rapid test. However it is preferable to screen all women for HIV during pregnancy when there is still time for adequate counselling.

Reducing HIV transmission during labour and delivery

3-4 Is there any need to isolate HIV-positive women during labour?

No. There is no need to isolate HIV-positive women before, during or after labour. However, there is a need for privacy when counselling these women.

3-5 Can the duration of ruptured membranes influence the risk of HIV transmission if ARV treatment or prophylaxis is not given?

Yes. Ruptured membranes exposes the infant to cervical and vaginal secretions. The longer the duration of ruptured membranes, the greater the risk of HIV in cervical and vaginal secretions getting into the uterine cavity and infecting the infant. The risk of transmission from mother to infant increases if the membranes have been ruptured for more than four hours, especially if the woman is not on ARV prophylaxis or treatment.

The risk of vertical transmission of HIV to the infant is increased if the membranes have been ruptured for more than four hours, without ARV treatment or prophylaxis.

NOTE Without ARV treatment or prophylaxis, the risk of HIV infection of the second twin is less than that in the first twin, as the second twin is exposed to maternal secretions for a shorter time.

3-6 Should the membranes be ruptured routinely in HIV-positive women?

No. The membranes should not be ruptured unless there is a good clinical indication. Artificial rupture of the membranes often results in the infant being exposed to vaginal and cervical secretions for more than four hours. Routine artificial rupture of the membranes must no longer be practised. This principle is also adhered to if patients are on ARV drugs.

NOTE There is no need to rupture membranes if labour progresses normally. However, with intact membranes and poor progress in the active phase of labour, rupture of the membranes should be considered. These patients need to be reassessed after a further two hours. Many patients will have progressed by then and be close to delivery. Those that have not progressed should be considered for Caesarean section.

3-7 How may the duration of labour influence the risk of HIV transmission?

In long labours there is a greater risk of transmission than in short labours, without ARV treatment or prophylaxis. As with the duration of ruptured membranes, the infant is exposed to HIV in vaginal and cervical secretions for a longer time with long labours than with shorter labours. It is believed that labour increases the risk of HIV crossing the placenta. Therefore prolonged labour should be avoided.

3-8 Is preterm labour more common in HIV-infected women?

Yes. The risk of preterm labour is doubled in women who are HIV positive.

3-9 May preterm labour increase the risk of HIV transmission?

Yes. The risk of HIV transmission is higher in preterm than in term infants, possibly because preterm infants have a more immature immune system and have fewer maternal antibodies. HIV in swallowed maternal blood or vaginal secretions may pass through the walls of their immature guts more easily. Even with ARV treatment or prophylaxis preterm infants still have a higher risk HIV transmission.

NOTE The presence of chorioamnionitis, which is a common cause of preterm labour, may also increase the risk of vertical transmission.

3-10 Does HIV infection in the mother cause intra-uterine growth restriction?

Intra-uterine growth is usually normal in HIV-positive women who are well nourished. However, poor fetal growth may occur if the mother is underweight and clinically ill with AIDS. Therefore,

HIV infection itself does not appear to cause slow fetal growth.

NOTE HIV-associated infections such as CMV may cause fetal infection and restrict intra-uterine growth.

3-11 Can Caesarean section reduce the risk of HIV transmission from mother to infant?

There is good evidence from the pre-ARV drug era that HIV transmission can be reduced by as much as 50% if a Caesarean section is performed, especially if it is done electively before the onset of labour. An elective Caesarean section prevents the fetus being exposed to cervical and vaginal secretions. As the infant does, however, still come into contact with maternal blood during the delivery, the risk of transmission is not eliminated. The risk of vertical transmission is not reduced much if a Caesarean section is done after the membranes have been ruptured. As a Caesarean section is expensive and requires the necessary staff and facilities, this is not a practical method of reducing the risk of vertical transmission in most poor communities. The benefit of an elective Caesarean section is much reduced if correct ARV prophylaxis or treatment is given to mother and infant. Therefore, Caesarean section is not used to reduce transmission in high HIV prevalence poorer resourced countries.

. . . .

Routine elective Caesarean section is not recommended to reduce the risk of HIV transmission to the infant.

. . . .

3-12 Is a Caesarean section dangerous in HIV-positive women?

Caesarean section has more complications in women who are HIV positive, especially if their CD4 count is low. The risks of wound sepsis and post-operative pneumonia are increased in HIV-positive women. Routine elective Caesarean section is, therefore, not recommended in HIV-positive women. Caesarean section should only be done if there are good clinical indications. Prophylactic antibiotics must be given to HIV-positive women who have a Caesarean section.

> NOTE If a Caesarean section is done in an HIV-positive woman, a spinal or epidural anaesthetic is preferable to a general anaesthetic as it carries a lower risk of pneumonia.

3-13 Can instrumental delivery increase the risk of HIV transmission?

Vacuum extraction, even with a silicone cup, always causes a small abrasion of the fetal scalp and should be avoided. Forceps delivery done with necessary caution will seldom result in skin injury and may be used for the correct indications.

. . . .

Vacuum extraction may increase the risk of HIV transmission to the infant.

. . . .

3-14 Should an episiotomy be done in HIV-positive women?

Whether a woman is HIV positive or not, an episiotomy should only be done if there is a good clinical indication. It should not be a routine procedure. HIV in maternal blood from an episiotomy may be swallowed and, thereby, may infect the infant during delivery. Healing of the episiotomy may also be delayed if the woman has depressed immunity.

3-15 Which women are most likely to transmit HIV to their infant during labour and delivery?

1. Women who did not receive ARV drugs or started ARV drugs late in pregnancy:
2. Women who become infected with HIV during their pregnancy as they have a high viral load
3. Women who have advanced HIV infection (AIDS) as they have a high viral load
4. Women with preterm labour and delivery
5. Women with rupture of the membranes for longer than four hours
6. Women who have prolonged labours

3-16 Are scalp clips safe in HIV-infected women?

No. Scalp clips damage the infant's skin and may allow the entrance of HIV. Therefore attaching scalp clips should not be done if the woman is HIV positive. Scalp clips should not be used routinely. However scalp clips could be used if clinically indicated in HIV negative women.

3-17 What is the value of vaginal cleaning with chlorhexidine (Hibitane) in reducing the risk of HIV transmission?

Wiping the vagina with 0.25% chlorhexidine (Hibitane) or povidone iodine (Betadine) does not reduce the risk of HIV transmission to the infant. Vaginal cleaning may reduce the risk of puerperal sepsis and neonatal sepsis. Routine use chlorhexidine cream for vaginal examinations is recommended.

3-18 Should all infants born to HIV-positive women be suctioned at delivery?

Unless infants are meconium stained or need resuscitation, they must not have their mouth and nose suctioned after birth as this may damage the mucous membranes and increase the risk of HIV infection. Sometimes, deep suctioning may cause apnoea in the infant. It may be helpful to wipe the infant's mouth and face after delivery to remove maternal blood and secretions. Suctioning of the mouth should not be done routinely on any infant.

Infants should not be routinely suctioned after delivery.

3-19 Should you clean infants born to HIV-positive women after delivery?

It may reduce the risk of HIV transmission if these infants are well dried and all the maternal blood and vaginal secretions are wiped off with a towel immediately after delivery.

These infants do not need to be bathed straight after delivery. Once dried they should be given to the mother if they are breathing well.

Antiretroviral prophylaxis in labour

3-20 Are antiretroviral drugs useful during labour to reduce the vertical transmission of HIV?

Women who have been on ARV prophylaxis or treatment during pregnancy do not need AZT and a prophylactic dose of NVP during labour as they have a low viral load with only a small risk of transmitting HIV during labour and delivery. They should continue their ARV drugs during labour. Most women would be on FDC and should continue taking a single tablet daily. Women taking ARV drugs will have a risk of HIV transmission during pregnancy and labour of less than 2%.

HIV-infected women who did not receive ARV drugs during the antenatal period must be given both NVP and AZT in labour.

Antiretroviral drugs given during pregnancy and labour will reduce the risk of spreading HIV to the infant to less than 2%.

3-21 How is AZT used prophylactically to reduce the risk of vertical transmission of HIV?

Oral AZT 300 mg should be given three-hourly during labour to HIV positive women who have not had ARV drugs during pregnancy.

3-22 How is nevirapine used prophylactically to reduce the risk of vertical transmission of HIV?

A single oral dose of NVP is taken by the mother as soon as possible after the onset of labour. If possible, the dose should be taken more than two hours before delivery to allow the drug time to cross the placenta to the fetus. NVP is absorbed rapidly. It is never too late to give single dose NVP during labour if women are on no ARV drugs. The dose of NVP for the mother is 200 mg (a single tablet). This is followed by NVP syrup to the infant, started as soon as possible after delivery. A single dose NVP taken during labour reduce transmission during labour by 50%.

● ●

All women not receiving ARV drugs during pregnancy must receive a single dose NVP plus 3 hourly AZT as soon as possible after the onset of labour.

● ●

A single dose of NVP to a woman in labour can result in HIV resistance to NVP and possibly EFV. Therefore a single dose of Truvada (TDF and FTC) should be given to the woman together with the single dose NVP or as soon as possible after the dose of NVP. This measure significantly reduces the risk of developing resistance against NVP.

3-23 Which risk factors are associated with an increased risk of transmission during labour even if antiretroviral drugs are used correctly for prophylaxis or treatment?

A high viral load remains a high risk factor

Preterm delivery and vaginal delivery are lesser risk factors

HIV in the puerperium

3-24 What complications may occur in the puerperium in an HIV-positive woman?

Infectious complications are more common in the puerperium in women with HIV infection. Therefore, these women must be closely observed for:

1. Infection of the genital tract (puerperal sepsis). This may cause secondary postpartum haemorrhage.
2. Urinary tract infection, especially acute pyelonephritis.
3. Pneumonia, especially in women who have had a general anaesthetic.
4. Wound infections, especially after Caesarean section, episiotomy or tubal ligation.

If any of the above occurs, appropriate antibiotics must be started immediately.

Preventing accidental HIV infection

3-25 Are nurses and doctors at risk of accidental infection when delivering HIV-positive women?

Yes. As vaginal and cervical secretions, blood and amniotic fluid may contain HIV. Healthcare workers can become infected by HIV via the following routes:

1. By needle-stick injuries or cuts during surgery
2. By exposing cuts or abrasions on one's hand to body fluids infected with HIV
3. By splashes into the mouth or eyes of body fluids infected with HIV

The risk of acquiring HIV infection by needle-stick injury or accidentally cutting one's finger during surgery is 1 in 300 without ARV prophylaxis while the risk of HIV infection after blood splashes or getting blood on cuts or abrasions is less than 1 in 1000 if ARV prophylaxis is not given. These risks are much reduced with ARV prophylaxis.

3-26 How can staff reduce the risk of becoming infected with HIV during a delivery?

In the absence of screening, all women should be regarded as HIV positive. Therefore, the following universal precautions should be practised during the labour and delivery of *all* women:

1. Gloves must always be worn during delivery.
2. Glasses, goggles or a mask with a visor must be worn if there is a risk

of blood or amniotic fluid splashing into one's eyes.

3. A plastic apron should be worn to prevent soiling of one's clothes.
4. Full precautions must be taken when handling needles or lancets. Both should be placed into a sharps container immediately after removal from the skin. Hollow and suturing needles must never be put down to be cleared away after completion of the procedure.
5. Great care must be taken to avoid pricking or cutting one's finger during surgery or while suturing an episiotomy.

3-27 What measures should be taken during a surgical procedure to reduce the risk of staff becoming infected with HIV?

1. All sharp instruments must be removed from the operating field as soon as they are no longer required. Sharp instruments must never be allowed to lie around.
2. A separate tray for sharp instruments is of value. The operator should then pick them up and put them down herself or himself.
3. A needle should always be held with forceps and not with one's fingers when suturing. A Bonney's forceps is ideal for this purpose as it has the necessary strength to grasp the needle.
4. Needles should always be safeguarded with the sharp point against the needle holder when not being used; even in between sutures while the knot is being tied.

Family planning for HIV-positive women

3-28 Why may an HIV-positive woman want family planning after delivery?

She may want to discuss family planning because:

1. A further pregnancy may speed up the progression of her disease, especially if she already has symptomatic HIV infection.
2. Of the risk of infecting her sexual partner during unprotected intercourse.
3. Of the risk of infecting any further children she may have with HIV.
4. She is worried that she may die of AIDS while her children are still young.

Family planning should be discussed with all women who have delivered. Women who are well and on ARV treatment should continue to use condoms because of the risk of becoming infected with another subtype of HIV or infecting uninfected partners.

3-29 What family planning advice should be given to an HIV-positive woman after delivery?

A permanent form of contraception may be advisable for HIV-positive women because of their reduced life expectancy that will result in their children being orphaned at a young age. The risk of transmitting HIV to each additional child also requires consideration. Postpartum tubal ligation should, therefore, be considered.

The methods of contraception usually offered to HIV-positive women are:

1. **Tubal ligation:** This is a very effective method but should not be done if the woman has AIDS because of the anaesthetic risk and the risk of post-operative sepsis. Vasectomy of the male partner is also an option in selected cases.
2. **Injectables:** medroxyprogesterone acetate (Depo-Provera or Petogen) and norethisterone enanthate (Nur-Isterate) provide reliable temporary contraception and are the contraceptives of choice. Both these contraceptives regimen remain effective irrespective of which ARV regimen are used.
3. **Intra-uterine contraceptive devices (IUD):** These devices can be used with safety, unless women are at risk of other sexually transmitted diseases. An IUD should not be inserted if women have AIDS (Stage 4 disease). Women who had an IUD inserted prior to their health deteriorating should continue with this method of contraception.
4. **Combined oral contraceptives (COC):** Effective if taken regularly. COC can be used with all ARV regimen except when ARV includes a protease inhibitor (PI). Women requiring a PI should switch to another form of contraception. LPV/r is a PI commonly used as a second line ARV regimen. COC may also fail if taken with antibiotics.
5. **Male or female condoms:** They are less reliable and must be used correctly every time intercourse takes place. Condoms also provide some protection against the risk of

spreading HIV infection and other sexually transmitted diseases.

6. **Abstinence:** This is the only certain method of preventing both pregnancy and the spread of HIV.

Emergency contraception with levonorgestrel 1.5 mg (2 pills) is effective but should not be used as a method of regular contraception. Lactational amenorrhoea (not ovulating during breastfeeding) is also effective if used with condoms during the first 6 months of breastfeeding if the infant is exclusively breastfed. However, not all HIV-positive women will be breastfeeding.

Whatever method of contraception is used, if there is a risk of spreading HIV, a condom must be worn.

3-30 How should you provide family planning for an HIV-positive woman?

1. Ask the woman what method she would prefer.
2. Decide whether there are any contraindications to this method.
3. If there are no contraindications, then this method should be used.
4. If there are contraindications, then more appropriate methods should be discussed.

Always give the woman information on the health benefits and the possible side effects of the method chosen. The need for proper compliance must be stressed. If both or only one of the sexual partners is HIV positive, a condom *must* be used during every act of intercourse.

Follow-up care of HIV-infected women

3-31 How should HIV-positive women be followed up after delivery?

If managed according to option B:

1. HIV-positive women who are healthy (stage 1 or 2 disease) with CD4 counts of more than 350 cells/µl during pregnancy must be reassessed in the puerperium. If they remained well FDC is stopped and they should be followed up with a CD4 count every six months at their local primary-care clinic.
2. Women who become ill with symptoms or signs of stage 3 or 4 HIV infection or have a CD4 count of 350 cells/µl or less must remain on lifelong ARV treatment and need referral for follow-up at their nearest ARV clinic.

If managed according to option B+:

1. All these women must remain on lifelong ARV treatment and need referral for follow-up at their nearest ARV clinic
2. If diagnosed to be HIV positive during labour or postpartum:
3. The mother need to be started on FDC, a CD4 count and serum creatinine requested and a follow-up date given for 1 week's time.
4. Good adherence and exclusive breast must be encouraged and supported.
5. Careful follow up during the puerperium for sepsis (uterus, breasts or wound) is important.

6. The infant also needs to be carefully followed up.

3-32 How should HIV positive women with TB or hepatitis B be managed?

All women must remain on lifelong ARV treatment irrespective of the CD4 count, if diagnosed with:

- Tuberculosis (i.e stage 3 HIV disease)
- Hepatitis B

Case study 1

An HIV positive G3 P2 woman, who is clinically well, with a CD4 count of 450 cells/ml, has been on FDC since 24 weeks gestation. At term she went in spontaneous labour, but progressed slowly from 4 to 5 cm cervical dilation, with membranes intact. The fetal condition was good. As the risk of HIV transmission was regarded as too high with rupturing membranes, a Ceasarean section was performed.

1. Do you agree with the decision to perform a Ceasarean section?

No, although there is evidence from the pre-ARV drug era that transmission can be reduced by as much as 50% if a Caesarean section is performed, especially if it is done electively before the onset of labour. She is already in established labour and the possible benefit of an elective Caesarean section has been lost.

2. How should she have been managed?

The membranes could have been ruptured and the woman reassessed following 2 hours. If there was still no progress a Caesarean section could be done. With normal progress of labour she will be close to a normal delivery.

3. Does a Caesarean section reduce the risk of transmission if a patient is taking ARV drugs?

The additional benefit of an elective Caesarean section is much less if correct ARV prophylaxis or treatment is given to mother and infant. Although the risk of intrapartum transmission is slightly reduced if an elective Caesarean section is performed, Caesarean section is not used to reduce transmission in high HIV prevalence and under resourced countries.

4. Is a Caesarean section dangerous in HIV-positive women?

Caesarean section has more complications in women who are HIV positive, especially if their CD4 count is low.

5. What complications could be expected if a Caesarean section is performed on HIV positive patients?

The risks of wound sepsis and post-operative pneumonia are increased in HIV-positive women. Caesarean section should only be done if there are good clinical indications.

Case study 2

An HIV positive G1 P0 woman is clinically well, with a CD4 count of 500 cells/ml and has been on FDC since 20 weeks gestation. At term she went in spontaneous labour and was admitted to a midwife obstetric unit for her delivery. She had already taken her FDC tablet for the day before arrival at the MOU. She had read up on the internet and is concerned about transmission of HIV to her infant during labour. The attending midwife decides to give her an additional single dose of NVP and to add 3 hourly AZT while in labour. Her membranes ruptured spontaneously at a cervical dilatation of 5 cm. She expressed her concern to the midwife that the risk of transmission had now increased.

1. What is the risk of HIV transmission during labour when women are healthy (stage 1 disease) and are on FDC?

Women who have been on ARV prophylaxis or treatment during pregnancy have a low viral load with only a small risk of transmitting HIV during labour and delivery. These women will have a risk of transmission during pregnancy and labour of less than 2%.

2. Will an additional single dose of NVP and 3 hourly AZT add any benefit to reduce HIV transmission?

Women who have been on ARVs during pregnancy do not need a prophylactic dose of NVP and AZT during labour. They already have a low

viral load and no additional benefit is to be gained by adding more ARV drugs.

3. What should the midwife explain to her patient regarding her concern following rupture of membranes?

She should explain that because she is on ARVs for a considerable time her viral load will be very low or may not be detectable. The risk of transmission, therefore, is not increased because her membranes ruptured.

4. What would be a correct policy regarding artificial rupture of membranes?

Membranes should not be ruptured unless there is a good clinical indication. Routine artificial rupture of the membranes must no longer be practised. This principle is still adhered to if patients are on ARV drugs.

Case study 3

An unbooked primigravida at term was admitted to a midwife obstetric unit following spontaneous onset of labour. She appeared healthy with an uncomplicated pregnancy. Her cervix is 3 cm dilated. She had never been tested for HIV. The midwife tells her that as she is already in labour she could only have an HIV test following her delivery.

1. Do you agree with the decision to postpone her HIV test until after delivery?

No, if a woman has not been screened for HIV during her pregnancy, she can still be screened during labour using a rapid test.

2. What would be the advantages of screening for HIV during labour?

Women diagnosed to be HIV positive in labour must receive single dose NVP during labour as well as 3 hourly AZT. The single dose NVP alone will reduce the risk of intrapartum transmission by 50%. The opportunity to reduce intrapartum transmission is lost if the HIV test is postponed until after the delivery.

3. Should you be concerned about resistance to NVP because the drug was given as a single dose?

A single dose of NVP to a woman in labour can result in HIV resistance to NVP and possibly EFV.

4. What measures must be taken to reduce the risk of resistance when using single dose NVP?

A single dose of Truvada (TDF and FTC) must be given to the mother together with the single dose NVP or as soon as possible after delivery.

5. How should the patient be followed up after delivery?

The mother need to be started on FDC, a CD4 count and serum creatinine requested and a follow-up date given for 1 week's time.

4

HIV in the newborn infant

Before you begin this unit, please take the corresponding test at the end of the book to assess your knowledge of the subject matter. You should redo the test after you've worked through the unit, to evaluate what you have learned.

Objectives

When you have completed this unit you should be able to:

- List the routes whereby infants can be infected with HIV.
- Correctly interpret diagnostic tests for HIV in infants.
- Use antiretroviral drugs prophylactically in newborn infants.
- Explain the risks and benefits of breastfeeding in HIV-positive mothers.
- Advise HIV-positive mothers on the choice of feeding methods.
- Manage infants born to HIV-positive women.

Introduction to HIV-exposed newborn infants

4-1 Can newborn infants become infected with HIV?

Yes. Newborn infants may become infected with HIV:

- During pregnancy when HIV may cross the placenta from a mother to infect her fetus.
- During labour and delivery when the infant may become infected with HIV present in cervical and vaginal secretions, and maternal blood.
- After delivery when the infant may become infected with HIV present in breast milk.

NOTE Rarely, the infant may become infected with HIV from transfused blood or by HIV-contaminated needles.

. . . .

Both the fetus and newborn infant can become infected with HIV.

. . . .

Infants cannot become infected by touching, hugging or kissing them. Neither can they become infected if vitamin K is given by intramuscular injection after they have been well dried.

The spread of HIV from a mother to her fetus or infant is called mother-to-child transmission (MTCT) or vertical transmission. Nearly all infants and young children with HIV infection have been infected by vertical transmission.

4-2 Do HIV-infected infants usually appear normal at birth?

Most infants that have been infected with HIV during pregnancy, labour or delivery appear normal at birth. Therefore it is not possible to decide by physical examination alone whether or not a newborn infant is infected with HIV.

....

Most infants with HIV infection appear normal and healthy at birth.

....

4-3 Does HIV infection cause congenital abnormalities?

HIV infection of the fetus does not cause congenital malformations. However, HIV-infected infants have an increased risk of having a low birth weight, especially if their mother is ill and underweight.

4-4 Should all infants born to HIV-positive mothers be suctioned at delivery?

Unless there is meconium-stained amniotic fluid or the infant needs resuscitation, these infants must not have their mouth and nose routinely suctioned after birth as this may damage the mucous membranes and, thereby, increase the risk of HIV infection. Routine suctioning should be avoided in all infants.

Diagnosing HIV infection in infants

4-5 Can the HIV screening tests commonly used on adults diagnose HIV infection in a newborn infant?

The diagnosis of HIV infection in a newborn infant is difficult as most HIV-infected infants appear to be normal and healthy at delivery. The HIV antibodies tested for in the ELISA and rapid HIV screening tests cross the placenta from mother to fetus. Therefore, if the mother's HIV screening test is positive then the infant's test will also be positive, whether or not the infant is infected with HIV. All infants born to HIV-positive women will have a positive HIV screening test at delivery. As a result, the HIV screening tests for adults is not useful in infants during the first months of life.

....

A positive HIV antibody screening test in the newborn infant does not necessarily mean that the infant is infected with HIV.

....

4-6 What blood tests are used to diagnose HIV infection in a young infant?

A DNA PCR test is routinely done at 6 weeks in all infants born to HIV positive women. If the PCR test is positive then the infant is infected with HIV. If the test is negative and infant is still being breastfed, the test should only be done again six weeks after the last feed of breast milk. A negative test, if the mother has formula feed her infant from birth, indicates an uninfected infant.

The results of the HIV tests in the infant, plus other details of management, must be added to the Road-to-Health booklet.

4-7 When can the HIV antibody screening tests be used to diagnose HIV infection in HIV exposed infants?

By 18 months after delivery all maternal HIV antibodies will have disappeared from the infant. A positive screening test at 18 months (a rapid test) indicates that the HIV antibodies are being produced by the infant and have not crossed from the mother during pregnancy. Therefore, two positive screening tests for HIV in an infant of 18 months or older indicate that the infant is infected with HIV. A negative screening test confirms that the infant has not been infected by HIV if the infant is no longer breastfeeding. This is a convenient time to screen these infants as they are attending a clinic for their booster immunisations.

All HIV-exposed infants with a negative polymerase chain reaction (PCR) test at six weeks should have a rapid HIV screen at 18 months.

4-8 Can the PCR test be used to identify when an infant became infected with HIV?

Yes, sometimes it may be helpful in identifying the time of infection. If the fetus is infected in early pregnancy then the PCR on the infant's blood will be positive at birth. However, if the infant only becomes infected in the last weeks of pregnancy or during labour and delivery the PCR will be negative at birth and only become positive by six weeks of age. The test will become positive more than six weeks after delivery in infants infected with HIV via breast milk.

Therefore the PCR test should be repeated six weeks after the last feed of breast milk has been given.

4-9 When do infants with HIV infection present with clinical signs of illness if they do not receive antiretroviral treatment?

1. Infants who are infected during pregnancy usually become ill in the first three months after delivery. They also rapidly progress to AIDS. Infants who are infected in the first half of pregnancy may present with signs of HIV infection as early as the first few weeks after delivery.
2. Infants that are infected during labour and delivery, or via breast milk, usually present much later and have a more slowly progressing illness. Signs of HIV infection in these infants usually present between six months and five years.

The earlier the infection with HIV the sooner the clinical signs of symptomatic HIV infection appear. The onset of symptomatic HIV infection can be prevented or delayed by ARV treatment.

If infants diagnosed to be HIV infected are started on ARV treatment while they are still healthy this will prevent them becoming symptomatic and developing the clinical signs of HIV infection.

4-10 At what age do HIV-infected infants die of AIDS?

Without treatment with ARV drugs, infants who present with AIDS soon after delivery usually die within the first three months of life. Most infants who present with AIDS in the first three months after birth are dead by six months of age without treatment while infants who present with AIDS after three months may survive beyond five years. The earlier the infection with HIV, the sooner AIDS develops and the worse the prognosis.

If infants diagnosed to be HIV infected are started on ARV treatment while they are healthy this would prevent most deaths of HIV infected infants and children.

4-11 When are infants at high risk for HIV infection during the antenatal period and during labour?

- Unbooked mothers diagnosed to be HIV positive during labour or postpartum
- Mothers that defaulted ARV prophylaxis or treatment
- Mothers with advanced HIV disease (stage 4)
- Mother known to have high viral loads
- Mothers that have been on prophylaxis or treatment for less than 8 weeks before delivery
- Mothers that give birth to preterm infants

4-12 When should a PCR test be done on infants who are at high risk of HIV infection before birth?

Ideally they should be screened with a PCR test before discharge from hospital after delivery. If diagnosed to be HIV infected and started on ARV treatment, these infants at high risk for early disease and death will remain healthy.

Preventing HIV infection in newborn infants

4-13 Can antiretroviral drugs be given to the infant after delivery to reduce the risk of HIV transmission?

Yes. If the mother is HIV positive, the infant should be given ARV prophylaxis after delivery (post exposure prophylaxis). This is most effective in reducing the risk of HIV transmission if the mother has been given ARV prophylaxis or treatment during pregnancy, labour and the first weeks of breastfeeding. However it will still reduce the risk of HIV transmission during labour and delivery even if the mother did not receive ARV drugs, if a rapid test is used to detect HIV-positive women during or immediately after labour or if she only started ARVs during the last 8 weeks of their pregnancy.

4-14 How should ARV drugs be given to the infant to reduce the risk of vertical transmission?

All HIV-exposed infants, whether the mother has received ARV treatment, ARV prophylaxis or no ARV drugs at all, should be given an oral dose of NVP after birth followed by a daily dose of NVP to the age of six weeks. The first dose must be given as soon as possible after birth, but within 72 hours of birth. However, if the mother has not been given any ARV drugs, the first dose of NVP to the infant must be within one hour.

Daily nevirapine can be stopped when the infant is six weeks old even in breastfed infants if the mother is on ARV treatment. In breastfed infants of HIV positive mothers who are not on ARV treatment, prophylactic NVP should be continued until one week after the last feed of breast milk.

* *

All HIV-exposed infants should be given a daily dose of NVP for six weeks after delivery.

* *

NOTE: If a mother was on ARV prophylaxis or treatment for less than 8 weeks before delivery the infant's NVP prophylaxis should be extended to 12 weeks and AZT syrup added for the first 4 weeks.

4-15 What is the daily dose of NVP for infants?

Most term infants will need 1.5 ml NVP from birth to six weeks. Thereafter the amount of NVP will increase as the infant gains weight. Dosages are shown in table 4-1.

HIV transmission in breast milk

4-16 What is the risk of HIV transmission from breastfeeding?

Most studies show that non-exclusive (mixed) breastfeeding for up to two years increases the risk of HIV transmission by an additional 15% if ARV prophylaxis is not given to the infant. The longer the mother breastfeeds, the greater is the risk of HIV transmission.

Mothers on ARV prophylaxis or treatment for at least 8 weeks before the onset of labour should have a very low or not undetectable viral load. The risk of transmission will be about 0.5% to 1% for the first 6 months of breastfeeding. This small risk continues if the mother breastfeeding beyond 6 months. Extended breastfeeding should be advised, as the health benefits of breastfeeding is more important than the small risk of transmission especially in poor communities.

Table 4-1 Daily dose of NVP for infants

NVP syrup 10mg/ml	Birth weight	Daily dosage	Quantity
	Less than 2.0 kg	First 2 weeks: 2mg/kg Next 4 weeks: 4mg/kg	0.2ml/kg
			0.4ml/kg
	2.0 – 2.5 kg	Birth to 6 weeks: 10mg	1.0ml
	More than 2.5 kg	Birth to 6 weeks: 15mg	1.5 ml

Mothers on Option B who are taking ARV drugs for prophylaxis must continue taking the ARV drugs until one week after the last feed of breast milk.

• •

The HIV transmission rate is lower with exclusive breastfeeding than with mixed breastfeeding.

• •

NOTE The reason why mixed feeding, with both breast milk and formula or solids, increases the risk of HIV infection might be because formula and solids can cause mild bowel inflammation. This may allow HIV in breast milk to pass into the bloodstream.

4-17 When can HIV be transmitted in breast milk?

HIV is present in breast milk. Even with an undetectable viral load HIV could be present in the white cells (leucocytes) in the breast milk. Therefore, infants can be infected with HIV at any time while they are still breastfed or receive expressed breast milk. Some infants may be infected by breast milk many months after delivery.

4-18 Can an infant be infected with HIV from another woman's breast milk?

Yes. An infant born to an HIV-negative mother may become infected with HIV if the infant receives breast milk from an HIV-positive woman. Breastfeeding another woman's infant, or using breast milk from anyone other than the infant's mother, is dangerous.

Pasteurised breast milk donated from HIV-negative women can be safely

used under strict control in newborn-care nurseries.

4-19 What factors may increase the risk of HIV transmission by breast milk?

• If the mother becomes infected with HIV while she is still breastfeeding, the risk of HIV transmission to the infant is as high as 50%. Therefore, breastfeeding women who are HIV negative should not have unprotected sexual intercourse.
• The risk is also increased in women who have a low CD4 count or clinical signs of AIDS.
• Cracked or bleeding nipples and mastitis or breast abscess increase the risk of transmission. Good breast care is, therefore, important for HIV-positive women who breastfeed.
• Milk from engorged breasts contains an increased number of white cells due to duct damage resulting in an increased the risk of HIV transmission.
• Sores in the infant's mouth, such as oral thrush, may increase the risk of HIV infection. HIV mothers should take their infants to a clinic for treatment if they notice oral thrush.
• Mixed feeding, with breast milk plus formula feeds or solids, increases the risk of HIV transmission.

• •

Good breast care and breastfeeding management are important to reduce the risk of HIV transmission.

• •

NOTE Inflammation or infection of the breast increases the number of leucocytes and the viral load of HIV in the milk.

Breastfeeding HIV-exposed infants

4-20 Should all HIV-positive mothers breastfeed?

There are both dangers and advantages to HIV-positive women breastfeeding. However, the advantages of breastfeeding are the lower risk of gastroenteritis, pneumonia and undernutrition, especially in poor communities. Therefore, many HIV-positive mothers from poor communities should be advised to exclusively breastfeed their infants for 6 months followed by extended breastfeeding after introducing solid foods. The final choice must be the mother's. She should be helped to make an informed decision.

Women should be advised to breastfeed unless the risk of HIV transmission in breast milk is greater than the dangers of formula feeding.

Several studies have showed that the overall HIV free survival in HIV-exposed infants from poor communities is significantly better when women breastfed compared to women who formula fed.

Women in poor communities should be advised to exclusively breastfeed for 6 months followed by extended breastfeeding when solids are introduced. The mothers on ARV prophylaxis must continue taking their ARV drugs until one week of completely stopping breastfeeding.

4-21 What breastfeeding information should be given to HIV-positive women?

All pregnant women must receive thorough infant feeding counselling during pregnancy. This requires four counselling sessions. During these session the importance of breastfeeding, the dangers of not breastfeeding and the addition of complementary breastfeeding following 6 months of age must be discussed.

The WHO suggests that women who choose to formula feed their infants should only formula feed if all the following are present:

1. Formula is available and affordable.
2. There is access to clean water and sanitation.
3. The mother is able to clean bottles and teats, or cups, safely.
4. The mother can mix formula correctly.
5. There is good primary care at local clinics.

Mothers who formula feed their infants should comply with the WHO criteria for safe formula feeding.

4-22 For how long should HIV-positive mothers breastfeed?

If women are receiving ARV treatment or prophylaxis and the infant's PCR was negative at 6 weeks, they should continue breastfeeding for one year. A mother of an infant confirmed to be HIV infected should be encouraged to breastfeed until 24 months.

4-23 How can feeding breast milk be made safer for an HIV-exposed infant?

Heat treatment of breast milk by pasteurisation kills HIV but also reduces the level of anti-infective properties, especially white cells. Home pasteurisation can be done as follows:

- Boil 450 ml water in a pot.
- Remove the pot from the heat when the water starts to boil.
- Place a glass jar, containing 50 to 150 ml expressed milk, into the hot water and allow to stand for 15 minutes.

Pouring boiling water from a kettle around the jar of milk standing in an empty pot can also be used. This method is particularly useful when caring for HIV-exposed preterm infants in hospital. Commercial pasteurisers are available but are very expensive.

4-24 How can feeding formula milk be made safer for any infant?

Cup feeding with formula milk is safer than bottle feeding as a cup is easier to clean with soap and water. After washing well, allow the empty cup to stand and dry. A feeding cup, which can be used to measure water,

mix formula and give a feed, is now commercially available. Cup feeding can also be used to give expressed breast milk to preterm infants who are not able to breastfeed yet.

It is easier and safer to clean a cup than a bottle.

All hospitals should use cups rather than bottles to formula feed infants.

NOTE Specially designed feeding cups can be obtained from Sinapi Biomedical (chrisd@sinapi.co.za or 021 887 5260).

4-25 Should HIV-negative women breastfeed?

Yes. It is very important that all HIV-negative women be encouraged to exclusively breastfeed their infants for 6 months followed by extended breastfeeding for as long as possible. Formula feeding in these mothers has many disadvantages, especially in poor communities where infection and undernutrition are common. All breastfeeding women should practise safe sex. These mothers need to screened again for HIV at the 6 weeks postnatal visit and at 3 months followed by 3 monthly screening while breastfeeding.

HIV-negative women should breastfeed their infants.

The many advantages of breastfeeding, especially exclusive breastfeeding, include:

- Breast milk provides infants with a balanced diet that meets all their nutritional needs.
- Breastfeeding reduces the risk of infections, especially gastroenteritis.
- It is cheap.
- Exclusive breastfeeding reduces the risk of becoming pregnant again soon after the delivery of the infant.
- It promotes bonding between mother and infant.
- It is usually socially and culturally acceptable.

4-26 When should women decide on the method of feeding their infants?

Whenever possible this decision should be made before or during pregnancy and not after delivery. This allows the woman time to consider all the advantages and disadvantages of breastfeeding. There is also time for counselling HIV-positive women.

The final decision must be made by the mother herself once she has been advised and she has discussed the options with family or friends. The medical and nursing staff must support the mother in whatever feeding methods she decides is best for her and her infant.

Formula feeding HIV-exposed infants

4-27 What advice should be given to a mother who decides to use milk formula?

- She must be sure that she can afford to buy adequate amounts of milk

formula, and that she will have regular access to milk formula.
- She must have access to a source of safe, clean water. Fuel (such as wood or paraffin) or electricity is needed to boil water to sterilise bottles.
- She must be taught to mix the milk powder correctly and not to make the milk too weak or too strong.
- She should use a cup, rather than a bottle and teat, to feed her infant as a cup is easier to clean, especially if facilities to sterilise bottles and teats are not available.
- If bottles and teats are used, they should be cleaned and sterilised before each feed.
- She should wash her hands with soap and water before preparing a feed.
- She should exclusively formula feed and not give a few breastfeeds as well.

If a woman chooses not to breastfeed, it is important that she is taught to formula feed safely.

4-28 Why may an HIV-positive mother decide to breastfeed even if she can afford milk formula?

- It may be traditional in that family or society to breastfeed.
- She may be afraid that the community will realise that she is HIV positive if she formula feeds.
- She may decide that the advantages of breastfeeding are greater than the dangers.

4-29 What can be done to help poor HIV-positive women obtain milk formula?

Sometimes poor women in urban areas meet the criteria for safe formula feeding but cannot afford to buy formula. For these women free milk formula could be provided on prescription. This requires prior arrangement within health facilities.

The state cannot provide free milk formula to all infants born to HIV-positive mothers in rural areas. Formula feeding for the first six months requires at least 40 x 500 g tins of milk, which is very expensive.

Providing free formula for HIV-exposed infants born in towns and cities may be a disadvantage if mothers are planning to take their infants back to rural areas soon after delivery. This could be disastrous for these infants if their mothers lose their breast milk and do not have access to free or affordable formula once they leave town. Equally dangerous is the practice of mix feeding in town so that they will be able to breastfeed when they return to the rural areas where free milk is often not available.

For these reasons the state has decided not to routinely provide free milk formula for infants of HIV positive mothers.

4-30 How could the state control the distribution of free or cheap milk formula to infants of HIV-positive women?

This problem does not have a simple answer. Formula milk could be dispensed by primary-care clinics and hospitals. If possible, milk should not be dispensed by those clinics where breastfeeding is promoted as this gives a confusing message to mothers. Every effort must be made to discourage the prescription of milk formula to HIV-negative women or women who do not know their HIV status. Breastfeeding must be promoted in these women.

Breastfeeding must be protected and promoted in HIV-negative women.

Care of HIV-exposed infants

4-31 Should all HIV-exposed infants be followed up after delivery?

Yes, as these infants must be correctly managed. It is very important that they are not lost to the health services after delivery.

4-32 How should infants born to HIV-positive mothers be followed up?

They should be followed routinely at the local mother-and-baby clinic for the first six weeks after delivery. During this time mothers must be encouraged to give their infants daily prophylactic NVP.

A PCR test should then be done at six weeks after delivery on all HIV-exposed infants:

- If the PCR test is positive the infant has been infected with HIV.

- If the test is negative and the mother has never breastfed or given breast milk, the infant is not infected
- If the test is negative but the mother has breastfed or given breast milk, the infant should be follow up and the test repeated six weeks after the last feed of breast milk. This is to assess whether the infant might have been infected late with HIV via breast milk.

It is cost-effective to use PCR testing as infants who are not HIV infected can receive routine infant care only. Infants with a positive PCR test are infected with HIV and need to be started on an appropriate ARV regimen.

A rapid screening test for HIV should be done at 18 months on all infants born to HIV-positive women, except those with positive PCR results. If the test is negative at 18 months, then the mother can be reassured that her infant is not infected, provided that she is no longer breastfeeding. If the test is positive, then the infant is infected.

HIV infection in infants

4-33 What is the management of infants infected with HIV?

- The mother must be counselled and informed about the diagnosis and management.
- Start antiretroviral treatment for life.
- Start co-trimoxazole prophylaxis.
- Provide multivitamin or vitamin A supplements.
- Give routine immunisations.
- Look for early signs of HIV infection.

- Ensure that the infant is well nourished.
- Monitor growth in the Road-to-Health booklet.

All infants under five years of age with HIV infection must be started on ARV treatment as the risk of symptomatic HIV and death is high in infants infected before, during or soon after delivery.

All infants under five years of age with HIV infection must be started on antiretroviral treatment.

4-34 What immunisation can be given safely to HIV-positive infants?

Infants born to HIV-positive women should receive all the routine immunisations.

It is important to immunise HIV-infected infants against these important infections, while they are still well. However infants with clinical signs of symptomatic HIV infection must not be given live vaccines (BCG, polio, measles, mumps and rubella). They can safely be given killed vaccines (DPT, Haemophilus and Hepatitis B).

Routine immunisations should be given to HIV-positive infants if they have no clinical signs of HIV infection.

NOTE In countries where TB is uncommon, BCG immunisation is not given to HIV-exposed infants until it is shown by PCR testing that the infant is not infected with

HIV. Only then is the BCG given as there is a risk developing local or generalised BCG disease in HIV-infected infants.

4-35 Why should co-trimoxazole prophylaxis be given to HIV-infected infants?

Prophylaxis against Pneumocystis infection and other bacterial infections should be given to all HIV-infected infants. Usually treatment is started at six weeks of age with co-trimoxazole syrup. Prophylaxis should be stopped if the PCR test is negative. Prophylaxis can usually be stopped at one year of age in infants on antiretroviral treatment. Co-trimoxazole (Septran, Bactrim, Purbac) syrup is started as a 2.5 ml dose every day. Adverse effects to co-trimoxazole are uncommon in young children. However, the drug should be stopped immediately if the child develops a generalised rash.

Prophylaxis against tuberculosis is usually not given routinely.

4-36 What is the importance of vitamin A supplements in infants with HIV infection?

In undernourished communities mothers may be deficient in vitamin A during pregnancy. As a result young infants may also be vitamin A deficient. A lack of vitamin A reduces the function of the immune system. Therefore, giving supplements of vitamin A to HIV-infected infants may reduce the risk of opportunistic infections and may slow the progress to AIDS. It is recommended that all HIV-infected infants receive 50 000 units of oral vitamin A at six weeks.

4-37 What are the presenting signs of HIV infection in a young infant?

- Failure to thrive with poor weight gain or with weight loss
- Severe or persistent oral thrush
- Generalised lymphadenopathy
- Hepatomegaly and splenomegaly
- Chronic, watery diarrhoea
- Recurrent infections
- Severe eczema or itchy papules

4-38 What infections are commonly seen in children with HIV infection?

- Gastroenteritis
- Severe bacterial infections such as pneumonia, meningitis, septicaemia, arthritis, osteitis or abscesses
- Recurrent, mild bacterial infections such as otitis media
- Severe herpes simplex infection
- Tuberculosis
- Severe chickenpox or measles
- Unusual infections often associated with AIDS, such as those caused by Pneumocystis. These are known as opportunistic infections. Pneumocystis usually presents as a severe pneumonia.

4-39 How is the clinical diagnosis of HIV infection confirmed?

1. A positive PCR test in infants less than 18 months
2. A positive rapid HIV screening test in infants at or over the age of 18 months

4-40 Who should care for an infant who is infected with HIV?

If possible they should be followed up regularly by a local primary-care clinic. However seriously ill infants may need to be referred to a special HIV clinic or to a hospital. All children with clinical signs of HIV infection who are not on antiretroviral treatment should be urgently referred as they need to start treatment. The aim is to identify those untreated HIV-infected infants before they have a damaged immune system and become seriously ill. It is important that there is good communication between the primary-care clinics and the HIV clinics in each health district.

First-line antiretroviral treatment in young infants is given with ABC (abacavir), 3TC and lopinavir/ritonavir.

4-41 What is an AIDS orphan?

One of the major tragedies of the HIV epidemic is that thousands of children are abandoned as orphans when their mothers die of AIDS. Many of these infants are not infected with HIV and yet are at risk of dying from malnutrition and neglect. Many HIV-infected mothers will die before their children are teenagers. It is the responsibility of families, the community and the state to care for these children. Often the child is cared for by a grandmother. Every effort must be made to keep AIDS orphans in their original community. This will require state subsidies and pensions.

If mothers are provided with antiretroviral treatment, many AIDS orphans can be prevented. Many of the infants who have lost their mother but are not orphaned, are not well cared for by the extended family who may already be caring for other infants whose mothers have died of AIDS. There are thousands of orphaned infants in South Africa.

Case study 1

An unbooked 18 year old G1 P0 woman is admitted at term in labour at a MOU. Her cervix is fully dilated and she deliveries within minutes. The mother and infant appear to be healthy. Both the initial and repeat rapid HIV tests done on the mother following the delivery are positive. The mother is regarded as at high risk for transmission and a rapid HIV test is done on a heel prick blood sample of the infant. The positive test on the infant is confirmed by a positive repeat test. No ARV prophylaxis is given to the infant who is thought to be already infected with HIV. The mother is started on FDC at discharged the next morning and the infant referred to the nearest ARV clinic to be started on ARV treatment.

1. Is this mother at high risk of transmitting HIV to her fetus during pregnancy and delivery?

The mother is unbooked and only diagnosed to be HIV positive following delivery. As she was not taking any ARV drugs during the antenatal period and labour she is at high risks of transmitting HIV to her fetus.

2. Can rapid HIV tests (antibody screening) be used to diagnose HIV infection in HIV exposed infants following delivery?

The HIV antibodies tested for in the rapid HIV screening tests cross the placenta from mother to fetus. Therefore, if the mother's HIV screening test is positive then the infant's test will also be positive, whether or not the infant is infected with HIV. All infants born to HIV-positive women will have a positive HIV screening test at delivery. As a result, the rapid HIV screening tests is not useful in infants during the first 18 months of life.

3. Could a PCR test be used to decide whether the infant was already infected with HIV at delivery?

Yes as a positive PCR test would indicate that the infant was infected with HIV during pregnancy.

4. Should post exposure prophylaxis be withheld if infants are thought to be at high risk for transmission?

No, all HIV-exposed infants, whether the mother has received ARV treatment, ARV prophylaxis or no ARV drugs at all, should be given an oral dose of NVP syrup after birth followed by a daily dose of NVP. The risk of transmission during labour is high if mothers are not on ARV drugs. This risk could be reduced considerably by giving NVP to the infant as soon as possible after delivery.

Case study 2

A 27 year old G1 P0 woman has delivered a healthy infant at term following an uneventful pregnancy. She is HIV positive with stage 1 disease and a CD4 count of 475 cells/ml. She was started on FDC at 20 weeks gestation and was compliant during pregnancy and labour. The mother is unemployed and lives in an informal settlement without electricity in her house and no clean water supply and proper sanitation. The mother says she chose to formula feed her infant as she does not want to take any risks with transmitting HIV to her infant with breastfeeding. She also states that she only wants to give the best to her infant.

1. Do you agree that formula feeding is the correct feeding option for this infant?

No, this mother does not comply with the criteria to safely formula feed her infant. Formula milk is expensive and she will not be able to afford formula milk. Access to clean water and sanitation is not present and it would be difficult for the mother to clean bottles and teats, or cups, safely.

2. What important information should be provided to the mother?

The advantages of breastfeeding should be explained to the mother. The overall HIV free survival in HIV-exposed infants from poor communities is significantly better when women breastfeed compared to women who formula feed. The risk of death due to gastroenteritis, pneumonia and undernutrition is significantly increased especially in poor communities.

3. What additional information regarding breastfeeding must be provided to the mother?

The mother must be advised to exclusively breastfeed her infants for 6 months followed by extended breastfeeding once she introduces solid feeds.

4. What is the mother's risk of transmitting HIV to the infant during pregnancy, labour and breast deeding?

The risk is low as the mother is healthy with stage 1 disease and she has been on FDC for last half of her pregnancy. The risk of transmission through breastfeeding is also low and would be about 0.5% to 1% for each 6 months of breastfeeding.

5. What ARV prophylaxis must be prescribed for the infant?

Give an oral dose of NVP after birth followed by a daily dose of NVP to the age of six weeks. The first dose must be given as soon as possible after birth, but within 72 hours of birth.

6. Would it be safe for the mother to stop the infant's daily NVP at 6 weeks?

Mothers on ARV drugs for at least 8 weeks prior to onset of labour have a very low if not undetectable viral load and NVP should be stopped at 6 weeks. Continuing with daily NVP beyond 6 weeks is only recommended for infants of breastfeeding mothers who only started on ARV prophylaxis or treatment during the last 8 weeks of their pregnancy.

Case study 3

A healthy male infant is born to an HIV-positive woman who has not taken her ARV drugs regularly. She breastfeeds as she cannot afford to bottle feed. At two months she brings her son to the clinic for the first time since delivery. The infant has not gained weight and has severe oral thrush and loose stools. On examination, generalised lymphadenopathy is noted as well as an enlarged liver and spleen.

1. What diagnosis would you suspect with the history of failure to thrive and oral thrush?

Severe thrush in an HIV-negative infant may result in poor weight gain as the infant finds sucking very painful. However, the combination of thrush, poor weight gain and loose stools in an infant born to an HIV-positive woman suggests very strongly that this infant has developed symptomatic HIV infection.

2. Would the clinical signs on examination support this diagnosis?

Yes. Generalised lymphadenopathy, hepatomegaly and splenomegaly all suggest that the diagnosis of AIDS is correct.

3. What blood tests could be used to confirm this diagnosis?

A positive PCR test would confirm the diagnosis of HIV infection.

4. If this infant developed signs of pneumonia, what additional diagnosis would you suspect?

The infant would probably have a bacterial pneumonia, Pneumocystis pneumonia or tuberculosis.

5. How can Pneumocystis pneumonia be prevented?

By starting co-trimoxazole prophylaxis at six weeks.

Case study 4

A preterm infant is born to an undernourished woman who was found to be HIV positive when screened at booking. She was not started on FDC and was only seen again when she was admitted in preterm labour and delivered a 1.5 kg infant one hour later. She did not receive NVP and AZT prior to delivery. NVP syrup was not given to the infant as the infant was preterm. The infant was given expressed breast milk by nasogastric tube for two weeks. Now the infant takes the breast well and at 4 weeks of age is ready to go home.

1. Why is this infant at an increased risk of HIV infection before delivery?

Because the infant was born preterm and the mother did not receive FDC prophylaxis. Neither the mother nor her infant have been given NVP. Her undernourished state could also be a sign of AIDS. This would suggest that she has a high viral load.

2. Do you agree with the choice of feeding method?

Yes, breastfeeding is the correct option. The milk must be pasteurised while in hospital followed by home pasteurization as the mother has not been on FDC for 8 weeks.

3. How should this mother and infant be managed?

Both mother and infant need to be assessed for ARV treatment. The mother needs to be started on FDC and the infant on daily NVP. The dosage of NVP syrup needs to be adjusted according the birth weight. A 1.5 kg infant should receive 0.2 ml/kg of NVP daily for the first 2 weeks followed by 0.4 ml/kg daily.

4. What is the danger of prescribing milk formula?

Women may be tempted to stop breastfeeding and use milk formula. It is very important that all women be advised and assisted to breastfeed. Prescribed milk may result in women not breastfeeding, even if they plan to move soon to a rural area where prescribed milk is not available.

5. What management should the mother receive?

She should be started on FDC. This will prolong her life, reduce the risk of HIV transmission in her breast milk and may prevent her young infant becoming an AIDS orphan.

5

HIV and counselling

Before you begin this unit, please take the corresponding test at the end of the book to assess your knowledge of the subject matter. You should redo the test after you've worked through the unit, to evaluate what you have learned.

Objectives

When you have completed this unit you should be able to:

- Explain the meaning of counselling.
- List the characteristics of a good counsellor.
- List the key principles and process of counselling.
- Provide counselling before and after an HIV screening test.
- Explain the advantages and disadvantages of taking an HIV test.
- Describe the possible reactions of a woman to a positive HIV test.
- Describe the legal rights of an HIV-positive woman.
- Counsel an HIV-positive woman who plans a pregnancy.
- Promote safer sex practices.

Introduction to counselling

5-1 What is counselling?

Counselling is a process by which a counsellor helps other people manage difficult situations in their lives so that they are able to find realistic ways to solve their problems. Counselling helps people to make their own choices rather than simply giving them advice or telling them what to do. Counselling empowers people to act on their choices and decisions, and provides them with an opportunity for personal growth and self-discovery.

Counselling is not simply about giving advice and instructions but rather about empowering people to solve their own problems.

5-2 What is a counsellor?

A counsellor is a person who helps people manage their own lives as effectively as possible. A counsellor is not someone who has all the answers and can solve other people's problems for them. Rather, a counsellor helps people make their own decisions in order to take the best course of action in solving their problems. It is important that the counsellor explains his/her role when a person is first given counselling.

5-3 What is the role of a counsellor?

The role of a counsellor is to:

- Be a good listener.

- Ask appropriate questions.
- Summarise what the person has said.
- Provide relevant information.
- Give emotional support.
- Help facilitate decision making.

5-4 What is the difference between counselling and education?

Although counselling includes the provision of information, it is much more than education alone. Counselling also provides emotional support and helps people to understand themselves and their problems. It also helps people to make their own decisions and to plan their future actions. Counselling always respects and maintains a person's confidentiality. Counselling requires active listening.

5-5 What is active listening?

Active listening includes hearing not only the words people say but also noting their body language and listening for the meaning behind their words. In order to understand what a person is saying and to respond appropriately the counsellor must become skilled in listening to people.

A good listener should:

- Stop talking. You cannot listen if you keep talking.
- Put the person at ease so that they can feel free to talk.
- Remove distractions. Close the door. Do not fiddle with notes or tap your pencil.
- Empathise. Try to put yourself in their place so that you can see the problem from their point of view.

- Be patient.
- Keep one's temper.
- Not argue or be critical.

Active listening is the key to effective counselling.

5-6 Who are counsellors?

A nurse, social worker, doctor or lay person can be a counsellor. A counsellor should have received training in counselling and be able to keep personal information confidential. The training of enough lay counsellors is one of the major challenges facing countries with high HIV rates.

5-7 What are the characteristics of a good counsellor?

A good counsellor should:

- Be a good listener and good communicator.
- Be respectful of the other person's feelings and point of view.
- Be kind, caring and understanding.
- Be non-judgemental (does not judge what is right or wrong).
- Be trustworthy and respectful of people's confidentiality.
- Be relaxed and calm.
- Be warm and approachable.

A counsellor should communicate confidence in a person's ability to make a good decision and to be able to cope.

5-8 What are the requirements of counselling?

- Sufficient time to reach out to the person and win their trust and confidence
- Accepting the person for who they are without judgement or prejudice
- Providing consistent and accurate information
- A place to speak privately
- Respect for confidentiality

5-9 What are some common errors in counselling?

Common errors counsellors make include:

- Talking more than listening
- Concentrating on facts not feelings
- Not accepting the other person's feelings or point of view
- Being judgemental
- Asking too many questions
- Avoiding silences
- Telling the other person what to do or how to feel
- Treating the other person like a child
- Assuming that they know what is best for the other person
- Giving their own opinions
- Using words and terms that the other person does not understand
- Allowing their own feelings to interfere in counselling
- Giving advice all the time
- Offering solutions before the problem has been explored
- Being impatient

A counsellor should do more listening than talking.

5-10 What are the key principles in counselling?

1. **Allowing people to make their own decisions**

People must make decisions for themselves. The counsellor's role is to facilitate this and not to make decisions for them. This is called client-centred decision making.

2. **Empowering people**

People should be encouraged to believe in themselves and their abilities. Counselling should help people to take control over their lives and set goals for the future.

5-11 What steps does a counsellor follow in providing counselling?

1. **Exploring the problem**

The counsellor should help people to:

- Define the actual problem
- Express their feelings

The counsellor can do this by listening actively, by asking appropriate open-ended questions (i.e. any answer is acceptable) and by allowing people to share their feelings.

2. **Understanding the problem**

The counsellor should help people to:

- Gain a clearer understanding of the problem
- Consider the options to solve the problem and decide on which one to follow

The counsellor can do this by explaining appropriate options and by encouraging people to look at the consequences of each option.

3. Taking action

The counsellor should help people to:

- Decide what steps to take to implement their decisions
- Overcome difficulties they may experience in taking action to solve the problem

....

Counselling should encourage people to believe in themselves and their abilities to make good decisions for themselves.

....

HIV counselling

5-12 What is HIV counselling?

HIV or AIDS counselling provides information and support to people with HIV infection to enable them to cope with their diagnosis and illness. It also helps them make the appropriate behaviour changes. Counselling helps people live positively and productively.

5-13 What are the goals of HIV counselling?

The main goals of HIV counselling are to:

1. Provide information
2. Provide emotional and psychosocial support
3. Give hope
4. Help people to improve the quality of their lives

5-14 What kind of information should be provided in HIV counselling?

The following should be discussed:

- The difference between asymptomatic HIV infection and symptomatic HIV infection (e.g. AIDS)
- The ways in which HIV can and cannot be transmitted
- Sexual behaviours which may transmit HIV
- Safer sexual practices that reduce the risk of becoming infected with HIV
- The increased risk of becoming infected with HIV if the person has another sexually transmitted disease
- The link between HIV and tuberculosis
- The HIV screening test
- The risk of HIV infection in pregnancy and breastfeeding
- The effectiveness of ARV prophylaxis and treatment

It is very helpful to give the person a pamphlet which explains these important points so that they can be read about at home.

5-15 How can HIV counselling help a pregnant woman?

HIV counselling helps a pregnant woman by providing emotional support as well as appropriate information so that she can make decisions and then act on these. Women may need help with the following issues:

- Whether to have the HIV screening test
- Options for practising safer sex
- Coming to terms with being HIV positive
- The risks of being HIV positive and pregnant

- The advantages of breastfeeding and the risk of HIV transmission to the infant
- How to tell her sexual partner of her HIV status

5-16 Which pregnant women need HIV counselling?

- Women who are offered antenatal HIV testing (screening)
- Women who decline HIV testing
- Women who are worried that they may be infected with HIV
- Women who are concerned that they may transmit HIV to others, including their infants
- Women who are HIV positive or have AIDS

All pregnant women in South Africa should be given HIV counselling when they first book for antenatal care.

5-17 Do women have a choice as to whether or not they are tested for HIV?

Yes. HIV testing (screening) may be offered to a woman but it is her choice as to whether she is tested or not. Women must never be forced to be tested. A decision to be tested should be an informed one which means that a woman should get counselling before the test is done. Verbal consent must be obtained before the HIV test is done.

Notes need be made in the maternity case records if women declined testing. Additional counselling sessions should be arranged for these women. Women often change their minds once more time is allowed and with additional counseling.

The decision to take an HIV test should always be the woman's own choice.

All pregnant women should be given provider-initiated HIV testing and counselling. HIV testing is done routinely unless the woman asks not to be tested. This practice of 'opt out' testing increases the number of women who agree to be screened for HIV. This makes HIV screening similar to that for other infections such as syphilis.

5-18 What counselling is needed when a pregnant woman is tested for HIV?

The implications of having an HIV test are potentially devastating. Women should be counselled before testing is done. This usually is provided in a group. Individual counselling is done following testing when results are given. Women who are HIV positive usually need further counselling as they face the life-changing implications of a positive test. Knowing that she is HIV positive may change her relationship with her present partner, and with any future partners. Good counselling is essential if an HIV screening programme is to be successful and accepted by the public.

Counselling for antenatal HIV screening

5-19 What counselling is needed before HIV screening?

The importance of pre-test counselling cannot be underestimated. This is where women are most likely to absorb information and identify people who will help them cope with their test results. The following topics should be discussed:

- Information about HIV infection and AIDS
- Why the HIV screening test is being offered
- The advantages and disadvantages of taking an HIV test
- The meaning of a positive and a negative result
- The woman's own risk factors for becoming infected with HIV
- Safer sexual practices
- The procedure for taking the blood sample and giving the results
- How long she will have to wait for the results
- The confidentiality of the result

The counsellor should provide an opportunity for women to ask questions. Ideally pre-test counselling should be provided on an individual basis. However, due to staff shortages, a pre-test information session, rather than individual counselling is usually given to groups of women.

An information session should always be provided before a person takes the HIV test.

5-20 What are the advantages of taking an HIV test?

- It may relieve the woman's anxiety and uncertainty about being infected with HIV.
- It could help motivate women with high-risk sexual behaviours to change these behaviours.
- It allows for planning in the pregnancy. For example, if a pregnant woman is found to be HIV positive she can make informed decisions about termination of pregnancy.
- It allows for better management of her pregnancy and delivery if she is found to be HIV positive. ARV prophylaxis greatly reduces the risk of the infant being infected with HIV.
- The woman can be encouraged to practise a healthier lifestyle.
- It will allow earlier diagnosis and treatment of HIV infection in both mother and infant.

5-21 What are the disadvantages of taking an HIV test?

If the test is positive:

- The woman may experience intense feelings of despair, anxiety, rage, fear, depression and loss.
- The woman may suffer from loss of self-confidence, self-imposed isolation and a sense of loss of control over her life.
- The woman may risk losing her employment with resultant financial difficulties should her employer find out that she is HIV positive. South African law protects women from unfair dismissal.
- The woman may not be able to obtain life insurance or take out a house bond. Again, people cannot be discriminated against because of their HIV status in South Africa.

- The woman has to live with the uncertainty of having to wait and see if and when she will develop signs and symptoms of AIDS.
- The woman may experience problems with relationships (love, family and friends) should she tell them that she is HIV positive.
- The woman may face stigma, discrimination, prejudice, blame and abandonment.

All pregnant women should be offered routine HIV testing.

5-22 How should the HIV test result be given?

The result should always be given in person, privately, gently and sensitively. The registered nurse or counsellor should give the result immediately as social chit-chat only heightens a woman's anxiety. With the rapid test, results should be available within 20 minutes.

5-23 What counselling is needed after a negative HIV result?

Usually the woman is relieved and pleased to hear the result. It is necessary to allow her time to express her feelings. The following topics should be discussed during the counselling session:

- The meaning of a negative result
- The meaning of the 'window period'
- Safer sexual practices for the future

During the window period, which lasts 2 to 8 weeks after the time of infection, the rapid screening test for HIV testing for antibodies may still be negative in spite of the fact that the person is infected with HIV.

5-24 What counselling is needed after a positive HIV result?

Counselling should always be offered at the time that the positive HIV test result is given. The discussion should be private and confidential. The counsellor needs to provide emotional support as well as explain the meaning of a positive test. Often the woman is too shocked and upset to absorb much information. It is vitally important that the woman is given an opportunity to deal with her feelings. This is not the time to provide too much information or to discuss her prognosis. One session is not enough and the woman should always be offered at least one follow-up session. The following guidelines should be used in post-test counselling sessions:

- Allow the woman time to absorb the news.
- Deal with feelings arising from the result.
- Identify the woman's immediate concerns.
- Identify a support system to support her emotionally, financially, socially and spiritually (family, friend, church).
- Discuss the problem of telling her sexual partner.
- Who else she will tell she is HIV positive.
- Repeat information provided in pre-test counselling. It is important to clarify the facts.
- Review safer sexual practices.
- Discuss a plan for medical follow-up.

- Give information about any local support organisations.
- Encourage the woman to ask questions.
- Remember the importance of encouraging hope rather than despair.
- Summarise and reflect on the woman's feelings at the end of the counselling session.
- Offer a follow-up counselling appointment.

. . . .

Information can only be provided once the counsellor has allowed the person time to express their feelings and concerns.

. . . .

Often one or more counselling sessions are needed after a woman is told that she has HIV infection.

Receiving bad news

5-25 What are common responses on being told that the HIV test is positive?

People may react differently to news of HIV infection. The person's personality, spiritual and cultural values often have a major effect on how they responds to bad news. The following are some common responses:

1. **Shock**

Often people are shocked when told that they are HIV positive. At this stage support is what is needed. They may sweat, feel dizzy and even feel that they are going to faint. Many will cry.

2. **Denial**

Often people go into a state of denial and believe that 'there must be some mistake'. This is a common response and results from feelings of anxiety and helplessness. It is not helpful to attempt to convince the woman at this stage that she should face reality. Rather, encourage her to talk about her feelings and anxieties and provide emotional support. This initial response is common and with effective counselling is usually short-lived. A good counsellor can help a woman to accept the result and begin to develop positive ways to manage her infection.

3. **Fear**

Most people respond to the news with a feeling of fear and panic. Many people with HIV infection fear abandonment and rejection by friends and family. They may fear pain, suffering, discomfort and dying.

4. **A sense of loss**

People who are HIV positive usually experience a tremendous sense of loss in their lives. The following are examples of these losses:

- Loss of control
- Loss of future dreams and hopes
- Loss of self esteem
- Loss of physical ability and health
- Loss of loved ones
- Loss of independence
- Loss of sexual relationships
- Loss of other relationships
- Loss of employment and income

5. Guilt

People may experience feelings of guilt over the manner in which they became infected with HIV, as well as guilt over other people they may have infected. This is particularly common for a woman who has infected her infant.

6. Anger

Some people with HIV infection experience episodes of anger for a variety of reasons:

- Anger that they have become infected
- Anger at the person who has infected them
- Anger because their life may be shortened

7. Depression

The feeling of helplessness and lack of control associated with the many losses experienced may lead to depression and even suicidal thoughts.

8. Anxiety

People with HIV infection have many anxieties:

- Anxiety about their own illness and death
- Anxiety about others finding out about their diagnosis
- Anxiety about being rejected
- Anxiety about family that will be left behind, especially children

These emotional responses are similar to those experienced when hearing about the death of a close friend or family member or being diagnosed with cancer.

Counselling women with HIV infection

5-26 How can a counsellor help a woman who is HIV positive tell her husband or partner about her infection?

Deciding to tell a partner is very difficult. Many HIV-positive women fear being rejected or abandoned. They are afraid of being blamed for what has happened and fear that their partner will tell others. Not telling a partner presents problems. The couple may then not be able to discuss whether or not to have children. They will also have trouble coping with illness or death. An unaffected partner may become infected after unprotected intercourse. Some suggestions for the counsellor are:

- Explore how the woman feels about telling her sexual partner and what her fears are. Women often have real fears that they will be assaulted or abandoned. A woman's physical safety is of top priority and it should be her choice as to whether to tell her sexual partner or not.
- Discuss her sexual partner's possible reactions.
- Do a roleplay with the woman.
- Offer to see her and her partner together if she chooses.

If the counsellor feels unsure as to how to handle a particular situation she should contact a local resource person, such as a social worker, clinical psychologist or priest, to obtain help.

5-27 Should a woman with a positive HIV test tell other people about her diagnosis?

The counsellor should help the woman to identify at least one person whom she trusts and who she would be able to turn to for support. She should reflect on the following questions:

- Who do I tell?
- Who would I not tell?
- What might happen if I tell people?
- How will my friends and family respond?

It is important that a woman does not rush into telling people before she has thought through the implications of doing so, such as losing her job or being rejected by people.

Encourage women to tell at least one person whom she can trust about her diagnosis so that she can get their support.

5-28 What should a counsellor do if a person with HIV infection asks her how long they have to live?

The counsellor should never attempt to make a prognosis of how long the person has to live, even if this question is asked. Rather encourage the woman to consider that she may have many healthy years ahead of her and to take good care of herself. Life expectancy and quality of life can be greatly improved with ARV treatment. Always give people hope.

5-29 Is an HIV-positive woman required by law to tell her employer of her HIV status?

No. There is no law requiring an employee (worker) to tell her employer (boss) what her HIV status is. This is her own choice and she should be encouraged to disclose this personal information only if her employer is likely to be fair and sympathetic.

The law does not require an employee to tell her employer of her HIV status.

5-30 What happens if a woman's employer finds out that she is HIV positive?

A person cannot be fired from their job simply because they are HIV positive. This is against the law (the constitution) in South Africa, and applies also to domestic and farm workers. The counsellor should encourage the person to contact her labour union for advice on how to manage this situation if the person faces dismissal.

5-31 How should an HIV-positive woman be counselled if she wants to fall pregnant?

Questions about pregnancy and HIV are among the most difficult to answer and should be handled with great sensitivity by the counsellor. Do not try to persuade the woman not to fall pregnant or you will drive her away from the health services. The counsellor should do the following:

- Explore why the woman wants to fall pregnant despite the risks involved.
- Explore what the effect would be for the woman if she did fall pregnant.

The counsellor should be able to help the woman make a wise and informed choice. These issues should be discussed in a kind, supportive and non-judgemental way.

5-32 Why may an HIV-positive woman want to fall pregnant?

- In many communities a woman's status depends on her ability to have children.
- She may prefer falling pregnant rather than telling her partner that she is HIV positive because of her fear of rejection, divorce or physical harm.
- Often women are prepared to take a chance because they feel that their infant will not be infected.
- They may want to leave behind a survivor if other children have died of AIDS.

5-33 What are the implications if an HIV-positive woman should fall pregnant?

The HIV-positive woman should consider:

- The possibility of having to care for a sick or dying infant
- What practical and emotional help she has to care for her child
- Who will care for the child if she and her partner die of AIDS
- Feelings of guilt, sadness and regret if her infant is infected with HIV

- Possible effects of pregnancy on her own health
- The risks associated with breastfeeding

With ARV prophylaxis or treatment during pregnancy, labour and breastfeeding the risk of transmitting HIV to the fetus can be greatly reduced. The risk will be less than 5%.

Safer sex counselling

5-34 What is safer sex counselling?

Safer sex counselling is not a series of commands to a woman. It is counselling which helps a woman to consider her risk of becoming infected with HIV or of passing HIV on to her partner. She also needs to make an informed choice as to how she will protect herself and her partner from infection.

Safer sex counselling should provide a woman with information and support to enable her to make choices that will protect her and her partner from becoming infected with HIV.

5-35 What options does a woman have to protect herself and her partner from HIV?

- Keeping to one HIV-negative sexual partner who she knows to be faithful.
- Using a condom every time she has sexual intercourse.

- Avoiding intercourse if she or her partner has another sexually transmitted disease.
- Getting early treatment for other sexually transmitted diseases.
- Practicing non-penetrative sex such as mutual masturbation.

Some sexual practices are safer than others. People are more likely to change their behaviour if they are able to choose which sexual practices they are happy with. Ask the woman to identify the most acceptable option for herself and her partner. Try to promote the idea that safer sex is a sign of caring for each other.

5-36 How does a counsellor promote the use of condoms?

- Discuss whether she has used condoms before and whether she has had good or bad experiences with the use of condoms.
- Discuss how she and her partner feel about using condoms.
- Ask what difficulties she has had in the past in using condoms. Discuss possible solutions to these difficulties.
- Discuss the benefits of using condoms. The risk of pregnancy and sexually transmitted diseases is reduced. The man will not ejaculate as quickly which will give her more pleasure during intercourse.
- Offer to role play in getting her partner to use condoms. This will give her confidence.

5-37 What are the benefits of joining an HIV support group?

A support group provides a person with HIV infection with the opportunity of meeting other people facing similar problems. They can support each other.

Support for HIV counsellors

5-38 Why may healthcare workers who counsel HIV-positive patients need emotional help themselves?

HIV counselling is extremely stressful work. Therefore, support and mentoring for all counsellors is essential. This helps to prevent burn-out and enables counsellors to continue to be effective. Stress management courses would also be very helpful.

Case study 1

A woman attends an antenatal clinic and is found to HIV positive. She asks the midwife whether she could continue having sex with her boyfriend. The midwife impatiently tells the woman that she deserves to have AIDS as she has had too many boyfriends. The midwife also lectures the woman on the dangers of being infected with HIV. The woman is very upset and refuses to return for further antenatal care.

1. What was the problem with the midwife's attitude towards the woman?

She was judgemental and impatient, and treated the woman as if she were a child. She also failed to answer the question as to whether the woman should continue to have sexual relations with her boyfriend. The midwife should have listened carefully to her story.

2. Why should a counsellor not lecture a patient?

The goal of counselling is to help people understand their problems in order to decide the best way to resolve them. A counsellor should not tell the person what to do. Counselling is much more than just education.

3. Should the midwife have informed the woman that her infant may become infected with HIV?

The midwife should have provided the woman with the information. However, this should be done with kindness and understanding. The midwife should have allowed the woman to ask questions and given her simple, honest answers. The woman needs to be told about the importance of ARV prophylaxis.

4. How would you have answered the question about further sex with the boyfriend?

The advantages and disadvantages of continuing the sexual relationship, both for the woman and her boyfriend, should have been explored. The woman would then have been able to make the best decision for herself. It would be important for the boyfriend to be screened for HIV.

5. Should a counsellor ever give advice?

Yes. Good advice may be given by a counsellor. However, this should only be given once the counsellor has listened to the person and explored the problem. Remember that the person being counselled need not necessarily take the advice. The counsellor should respect this decision and support the person even if her advice is refused.

6. Are you surprised that the woman refuses further antenatal care?

No. Her trust in the care of the midwife has been broken. She was not given the support that she needed, and she was treated in an unkind way.

7. What can be done to correct the situation?

A staff member with counselling skills needs to make an appointment for the woman to come and see her or visit the woman at her home. She should provide her with the information and support she needs, and gently persuade her to attend the antenatal clinic again.

Case study 2

A group of pregnant women are being counselled by a midwife in the waiting area of an primary care antenatal care clinic before being tested for HIV. They are instructed that all pregnant women must take the test. As the midwife has a busy clinic ahead, she briefly tells the women that infants can become infected through breastfeeding, and that they should, therefore, not breastfeed if they are HIV positive.

1. Is counselling always necessary before an HIV test?

Yes. It is essential that a woman understands the advantages and disadvantages of HIV screening before having an HIV test.

2. Should counselling before HIV testing be given to patients as a group?

Whenever possible counselling should be given on a one-to-one basis. However, due to staff shortages, information most often has to be given to a group of women.

3. Does counselling have to be given by a doctor or midwife?

No, lay people can be trained to become very skilled counsellors. Most of the antenatal counselling in South Africa is given by lay counsellors.

4. Do all pregnant women have to take an HIV test?

No. Women do not have to take an HIV test. HIV screening is voluntary. However, 'opt out' routine HIV testing is provided in South Africa. A note needs to be made in the maternity case record that the woman declined HIV screening. In addition further counselling sessions need to be scheduled for the woman.

5. Why was the pre-test counselling inadequate?

The woman should not have been told that they have to take the test. Only the risk to the infant while breastfeeding was mentioned and no explanation was provided. Incorrect information regarding infant feeding was given. There are many other important subjects that must be discussed. The midwife was in a hurry and, therefore, there was no time for the women to ask questions. Information should have been provided so that they could make an informed choice.

Case study 3

A pregnant woman is told that her HIV test is positive. This is her second pregnancy. She insists that the result must be incorrect. When the midwife assures her that her test is indeed positive, she becomes very distressed and cries. Later she threatens the counsellor. Before she leaves the clinic, she asks whether she should tell her boyfriend the news.

1. Is it common for a person to refuse to accept a positive HIV result?

Yes. Shock and denial are often the first responses to bad news. With time and explanation the result is usually accepted.

2. How can a counsellor help a woman who is very upset after receiving bad news?

By being kind, understanding and supportive. Allow the woman to speak about her fears and anxieties.

3. Why was the woman aggressive towards the counsellor?

Some people respond to bad news with anger and aggression. They are angry that they are infected with HIV, and angry with the person who infected them. They may also be angry with the person who gives them the bad news. Anger usually quickly turns to guilt and depression. A counsellor should not react negatively to a person who feels angry, but encourage her to talk about her feelings.

4. Should she tell her boyfriend?

She needs to speak to the counsellor about his possible responses and how these will affect her life and that of her child. Women often do not pass on the news as they are afraid of rejection, anger and possibly violence. Each woman has to make her own decision. She should be encouraged to tell one, trusted friend.

Case study 4

A young woman with a two-year-old child returns to an ARV clinic for a 6 monthly check-up. She was found to be HIV positive when screened during the antenatal period. She told her employer that she was positive, and as a result she lost her job as a waitress. At present she has a new boyfriend and is considering falling pregnant again.

1. Does she need further counselling?

Many HIV-positive women need further counselling as new problems arise. She has lost her job, has a new boyfriend and is planning to fall pregnant again. All of these require further counselling.

2. Did her employer have the legal right to dismiss her?

No. An employee cannot be fired from her job simply because she is HIV positive. A labour union could be contacted to find out more about what to do regarding this matter.

3. Should she have another child?

Whatever the opinion of the counsellor, the young woman needs to be helped to make the best decision for herself, her child and her boyfriend. She should then be supported in her decision.

4. How can she protect her boyfriend from HIV infection?

Safe sex counselling must be provided as both she and her boyfriend should practice safer sex. Also explore her feelings about telling her boy friend that she is HIV infected. If she decides not to fall pregnant again, she should use a condom every time she has sexual intercourse.

Tests

Test 1: Introduction to perinatal HIV

Please choose the one, most correct answer to each question or statement.

1. What is HIV?

a. A retrovirus
b. A herpes virus
c. The human influenza virus
d. The cause of syphilis

2. What is AIDS?

a. A serious illness caused by a virus
b. A fatal disease whose cause is unknown
c. A common cause of abnormal sexual behaviour
d. An acute bacterial illness transmitted by sexual intercourse

3. You can become infected with HIV by:

a. Sharing a cup or plate
b. Social kissing
c. Unprotected sexual intercourse
d. Donating blood

4. Which body secretions may contain large amounts of HIV?

a. Urine
b. Stool
c. Blood
d. Saliva

5. Which blood tests are usually used to screen adults for HIV infection?

a. VDRL or RPR
b. ELISA or rapid test
c. PCR or p24 antigen
d. TPHA or FTA

6. Common features of the acute illness following HIV infection (acute seroconversion illness) are:

a. Blood and protein in the urine
b. Vaginal or urethral discharge
c. Anaemia and jaundice
d. Sore throat and rash

7. Usually the latent phase between the time of HIV infection and developing AIDS in adults is:

a. Two to four weeks
b. Six to 12 months
c. One to five years
d. Five to 15 years

8. What are the most common signs of symptomatic HIV infection in adults?

a. Weight loss and chronic diarrhoea
b. Oedema and heart failure
c. Cyanosis and wheezing
d. Jaundice and abdominal distension

9. What is an important opportunistic infection in AIDS?

a. Syphilis

b. Pneumocystis
c. Measles
d. Influenza

10. AIDS can be cured?

a. Always
b. Often
c. Sometimes
d. Never

11. What other disease can increase the risk of becoming infected with HIV?

a. Tuberculosis
b. Kaposi's sarcoma
c. Syphilis
d. Influenza

12. HIV is infectious:

a. Only during the first few weeks after infection
b. During the latent phase when the patient feels well
c. Only when the signs of AIDS appear
d. At any time after infection

13. How does HIV damage the immune system?

a. By destroying CD4 lymphocytes
b. By reducing the number of CD8 lymphocytes
c. By lowering the levels of antibody
d. By interfering with the function of the polymorphs

14. What type of drugs are nevirapine (NVP) and efavirenz (EFV)?

a. Antibiotics
b. Protease inhibitors
c. Non-nucleotide reverse transcriptase inhibitors

d. Nucleoside and nucleotide reverse transcriptase inhibitors

15. What is a common minor side effect of zidovudine (AZT)?

a. Tinnitus (ringing sound in the ears)
b. Sore throat
c. Nausea and vomiting
d. Rash

16. What drug is commonly used to prevent an opportunistic infection?

a. Penicillin
b. Co-trimoxazole (Septran, Bactrim, Purbac)
c. Nystatin (mycostatin)
d. Streptomycin

17. What is the management of a patient with AIDS?

a. Management does not alter the course of the disease and, therefore, is not recommended.
b. These patients should not be treated as it is too expensive.
c. Management with ARV drugs can make a big difference to the quality of the patient's life.
d. HIV patients should be sent home to die quickly as treatment only prolongs their suffering.

18. How can healthcare workers reduce the risk of HIV infection?

a. By refusing to care for AIDS patients
b. By washing their hands after touching patients with HIV infection
c. By wearing masks and gowns when caring for patients with HIV infection
d. By adopting universal precautions

19. What is the correct handling of sharps to avoid accidental injury?

a. Use a sharps container
b. Always resheath a needle after it has been used
c. Always wipe a needle with alcohol after it has been used
d. Only clear away the needle after the procedure has been completed

20. What prophylaxis should be given to a healthcare worker after an accidental needle-stick injury when collecting blood from an HIV-positive patient?

a. Penicillin should be given immediately
b. Truvada and Aluvia should be started within two hours
c. Hepatitis A vaccine should be given within 72 hours
d. Co-trimoxazole

Test 2: HIV in pregnancy

Please choose the one, most correct answer to each question or statement.

1. What percentage of pregnant women in South Africa are infected with HIV?

a. Less than 5%
b. Between 5% and 10%
c. About 30%
d. More than 50%

2. Which test can be used to screen pregnant women for HIV?

a. CD4 count
b. Viral load
c. VDRL test
d. Rapid test

3. What is the risk of transmission of HIV from a mother to her fetus during pregnancy, labour and vaginal delivery if they do not have ARV prophylaxis?

a. Less than 10%
b. Between 10 and 30%
c. Between 30 and 50%
d. More than 50%

4. The following women are at an increased risk of transmitting HIV to their fetus:

a. Women who become infected with HIV during the pregnancy
b. Women who are infected with HIV a few years before they fall pregnant
c. Women who are pregnant for the first time
d. Women who have had previous pregnancies

5. Which women at an antenatal clinic should be counselled about the benefits of HIV screening?

a. Only women who request an HIV test
b. All women
c. Only unmarried women
d. Only women with syphilis

6. How should women be told the result of the screening test?

a. It is best to inform them by post as this is the most private way to give them the results.
b. They should be told in small groups so that they can give each other emotional support.
c. They should be individually counselled and told the results.
d. Only HIV-positive women should be told their test result.

7. What precautions should a pregnant woman take to avoid becoming infected with HIV?

a. Use a diaphragm.
b. Douche with water after sexual intercourse.
c. Use a condom.
d. There is no need to take precautions once she is pregnant.

8. What effect may asymptomatic HIV infection have on pregnancy?

a. HIV has no effect on pregnancy.
b. Pneumonia is more common.
c. Placenta praevia is more common.
d. Gestational proteinuric hypertension (GPH or PET) is more common.

9. Which one of the following procedures may increase the risk of HIV transmission during pregnancy?

a. Amniocentesis
b. Vaginal examination
c. Abdominal palpation
d. Taking a cervical cytology (PAP) smear

10. Which ARV drug is used to reduce the risk of HIV transmission to the fetus?

a. Co-trimoxazole
b. INH
c. FDC
d. Tetracycline

11. How may ARV drugs reduce the risk of vertical transmission?

a. By inducing labour early
b. By preventing fetal distress
c. By reducing the viral load
d. By treating syphilis

12. Providing lifelong ARV treatment to all pregnant women who are HIV positive is called:?

a. WHO option A
b. WHO option B
c. WHO option B+
d. WHO option C

13. There is a concern about a possible association with congenital abnormalities and which of the following ARV drugs, when used in the first trimester?

a. AZT
b. TDF
c. FTC
d. EFV

14. Which statement regarding the use of multivitamins by pregnant woman who is HIV positive is true?

a. They will not reduce the risk of vertical transmission of HIV.
b. They will reduce the risk of vertical transmission by 50%.
c. They will block the effects of most ARV drugs.
d. They will lower the CD4 count.

15. Is AIDS an important cause of maternal death in South Africa?

a. It is not a cause of maternal death.
b. It is an uncommon cause of maternal death.
c. In the future it may become an important cause of maternal death.
d. It is the most common cause of maternal death.

16. May pregnancy cause a more rapid progression of HIV infection from stage 3 to 4?

a. Yes

b. Only in older women
c. Only with a twin pregnancy
d. No

17. Which opportunistic infection is most common in pregnant women with stage 3 HIV infection?

a. Oesophageal candidiasis
b. Pulmonary tuberculosis
c. Pneumocyctis pneumonia
d. Cryptococcal meningitis

18. Prophylactic co-trimoxazole is given to pregnant women with AIDS to prevent:

a. Oesophageal candidiasis
b. Tuberculosis
c. Herpes zoster
d. Pneumocystis pneumonia

19. What is an important side effect of TDF?

a. Anaemia
b. Severe skin rash
c. Renal failure
d. Bad dreams

20. Which drugs are used to treat tuberculosis during pregnancy in women who are HIV positive?

a. Anti-TB drugs should only be started after the infant is born
b. Rifampicin, INH, pyrizinamide and ethambutol (Rifafour)
c. Rifampicin, INH, pyrizinamide only
d. Rifampicin alone

Test 3: HIV during labour and delivery

Please choose the one, most correct answer to each question or statement.

1. What is the chance of mother-to-infant transmission of HIV during labour and vaginal delivery if the woman is not receiving antiretroviral prophylaxis?

a. 5%
b. 15%
c. 25%
d. 50%

2. Can HIV infection be diagnosed for the first time during labour?

a. Yes, by using a rapid screening test
b. Only if the labour lasts longer than 12 hours as the test takes many hours to perform
c. Only if the woman has clinical signs of AIDS
d. No

3. During labour, women who are HIV positive should be:

a. Isolated in a single ward and barrier nursed
b. Cared for with other women in the general labour ward
c. Cared for in a clinic only and not admitted to a hospital if complications develop
d. Always be cared for at home where they cannot infect other patients

4. In women who are HIV positive, the membranes should:

a. Be ruptured as soon as possible to speed up the labour
b. Be ruptured when the cervix reaches 4 cm dilatation
c. Only be ruptured when the cervix is 8 cm dilated
d. Not be artificially ruptured unless there is a good clinical indication

5. In women with HIV infection:

a. The risk of preterm labour is the same as in HIV-negative women
b. The risk of preterm labour is doubled
c. The risk of preterm labour is reduced
d. Preterm labour is rare

6. The risk of vertical transmission is increased in:

a. Preterm labour
b. Post-term labour
c. Term labour
d. Rapid labours

7. Does HIV infection in a well-nourished mother cause intra-uterine growth restriction?

a. Usually it does
b. Usually it does not
c. Only if the mother is receiving zidovudine (AZT)
d. Only if chorioamnionitis is present

8. The following procedure may reduce the risk of mother-to-infant transmission of HIV, especially if ARV prophylaxis has not been used:

a. Elective Caesarean section
b. A Caesarean section while in labour
c. An episiotomy
d. Vacuum extraction

9. Caesarean section in HIV-positive women:

a. Increases the risk of maternal wound sepsis
b. Decreases the risk of maternal pneumonia in the puerperium
c. Increases the risk of bacterial infection in the infant
d. Decreases the risk of hyaline membrane disease in the infant

10. In HIV-positive women, an episiotomy should:

a. Be done routinely to shorten the second stage of labour
b. Should never be done because it does not heal
c. Should only be done if there is a good clinical reason as it may increase the risk of vertical transmission to the infant
d. Only be done by a doctor

11. Which HIV-positive women are at greatest risk of transmitting the virus to their infant?

a. Women in the latent phase of the infection
b. Women who have clinical signs of advanced HIV disease
c. Women who have short labours
d. Women who have not transmitted HIV to their previous children

12. The following procedure may reduce the risk of mother-to-infant transmission of HIV during labour and delivery by 50% if an unbooked mother is diagnosed to be HIV positive when admitted in labour:

a. Giving the infant intramuscular vitamin K after delivery
b. Active management of the third stage of labour
c. Speed up labour with an oxytocin infusion
d. Giving the mother a single dose of NVP

13. Vaginal wiping with chlorhexidine during labour in HIV-positive women may:

a. Reduce the risk of HIV transmission
b. May reduce the risk of puerperal sepsis and neonatal sepsis
c. Cause inflammation and increase the risk of HIV transmission
d. Reduce the risk of meconium aspiration

14. After delivering the infant of an HIV-positive woman:

a. The infant's mouth should be well suctioned.
b. The infant should not be fed for 12 hours.
c. The infant should be well dried.
d. The infant should not be given to the mother for at least six hours.

15. During labour and delivery mothers on FDC should:

a. Receive a single dose of NVP
b. Continue with daily FDC
c. All ARV drugs should temporarily be stopped and only restarted after delivery
d. Receive 3 hourly AZT

16. What drugs should be given to women at the same time or after delivery if they receive a single dose of nevirapine in labour?

a. AZT and 3TC
b. TDF and FTC (Truvada)
c. Nevirapine and AZT
d. Lopinavir and ritonavir

17. Which risk factor is associated with an increased risk of HIV transmission during labour even if ARV drugs are used correctly for prophylaxis or treatment?

a. Elective Caesarean section
b. Posterm delivery
c. Male infant
d. A high viral load

18. How can staff reduce the risk of becoming infected with HIV themselves during the management of labour?

a. They should not perform vaginal examinations.
b. They should not rupture the membranes.
c. They should wear gloves.
d. They should be immunised against HIV.

19. How can staff reduce the risk of becoming infected themselves with HIV during Caesarean section or episiotomy repair?

a. Needles should always be held with forceps.
b. The patient must be washed with chlorhexidine.
c. Hands should be washed after the procedure is completed.
d. Needles must be hand held whenever possible.

20. What form of family planning will reduce the risk of spreading HIV to a sexual partner?

a. Tubal ligation
b. Injectables, such as Depo-Provera
c. Male or female condoms
d. Oral contraceptives

Test 4: HIV in the newborn infant

Please choose the one, most correct answer to each question or statement.

1. How may HIV be transmitted from a woman to her newborn infant?

a. By touching the infant
b. By kissing the infant
c. By breastfeeding the infant
d. By hugging the infant

2. HIV infection during pregnancy commonly causes:

a. Stillbirth
b. Congenital abnormalities
c. Clinical signs of HIV infection in the infant at birth
d. No sign of infection in the newborn infant

3. HIV infection in the newborn infant is confirmed if the following test is positive:

a. TPHA
b. VDRL
c. Rapid HIV test
d. PCR

4. When can a rapid test be used to diagnose HIV infection in an infant?

a. At 18 months of age
a. At one year of age
b. At three months of age
c. At birth

5. Infants who are infected with HIV during labour or delivery usually present with clinical signs of infection:

a. During the first month of life
b. Between one and three months of age

c. Between three and six months of age
d. After six months of age

6. Which HIV exposed infants should have NVP at birth?

a. All HIV exposed infants
b. Only if the mother did not receive ARV prophylaxis or treatment
c. Only if maternal ARV prophylaxis or treatment started in the last month of pregnancy
d. Only if the mother received ARV prophylaxis or treatment from 14 weeks

7. What is the added risk of HIV infection if the mother and infant are taking ARV drugs correctly and exclusively breastfeeding for 6 months?

a. 10%
b. 5%
c. 0.5% to 1%
d. 0%

8. HIV can be transmitted through the breast milk:

a. At any time that the infant is still breastfed
b. Only during the first few days when the mother is producing colostrum
c. Only while the infant is exclusively breastfed
d. Only if the infant has oral thrush

9. What factors may increase the risk of HIV transmission by breast milk?

a. Prolonged suckling during a feed
b. Engorged breasts
c. Puerperal sepsis with fever
d. A breast abscess with the previous infant

10. What method of infant feeding should be used by HIV-positive mothers?

a. They should all exclusively breastfeed for three months followed by rapid weaning
b. They should only feed their infants with formula milk.
c. They should exclusively breastfeed for six months followed by extended breastfeeding once solids are started
d. They should supplement breastfeeding with formula milk

11. For how long should a healthy HIV-positive woman on ARV prophylaxis breastfeed if the infant's PCR at 6 weeks was negative?

a. They should exclusive breastfeed followed by rapid weaning at 3 months
b. They should exclusive breastfeed followed by rapid weaning at 6 months
c. They should continue breastfeeding followed by slow weaning at 9 months
d. They should continue breastfeeding for one year

12. How can HIV be killed in expressed breast milk?

a. By keeping the milk in a fridge for 24 hours
b. By pasteurisation
c. By allowing the milk to stand at room temperature for 6 hours
d. By adding multivitamin drops to the milk

13. Expressed breast milk to preterm infants who are not able to breastfeed yet should be given by:

a. Cup if possible
b. Nasogastric tube until term
c. Bottle when they are old enough to suck
d. Breast milk should not given to preterm infants as they are at high risk of becoming infected

14. What feeding advice should be given to HIV-negative women?

a. They should not breastfeed as they may still become infected with HIV.
b. They should only breastfeed for three months.
c. They should breastfeed for as long as possible.
d. It does not matter whether they breast or formula feed.

15. If the PCR test of breastfeeding infant is negative at 6 weeks, when should a repeat test be done?

a. Following a further 3 months of breastfeeding
b. At 6 months
c. Six weeks after the last feed of breast milk
d. At 18 months

16. Which immunisations should be given to well infants born to HIV-positive women?

a. All routine immunisations
b. Only dead vaccines such as DPT
c. Only BCG
d. None at all

17. What prophylactic drug should be given to all HIV-infected infants?

a. Penicillin

b. Isoniazid (INH)
c. Co-trimoxazole (Septran, Bactrim, Purbac)
d. Nystatin (Mycostatin)

18. What are the presenting signs of symptomatic HIV infection in a young infant?

a. They often develop cancer
b. Failure to thrive or weight loss
c. Vomiting and abdominal distension
d. Oedema and excessive weight gain

19. What infections are commonly seen in infants with HIV infection?

a. Measles
b. Gastroenteritis
c. Syphilis
d. Toxoplasmosis

20. Who should follow up a well infant born to an HIV-positive mother?

a. A paediatrician at a level II or III hospital
b. A doctor at a special HIV clinic
c. A medical officer at a district hospital
d. A registered nurse at a primary-care clinic

Test 5: HIV and counselling

Please choose the one, most correct answer to each question or statement.

1. Counselling is a process whereby a counsellor:

a. Tells people what to do
b. Educates people
c. Helps people make their own decisions
d. Judges people

2. The key to good counselling is:

a. Concentrating on facts and not feelings
b. Being a good listener and communicator
c. Assuming that you know what is best for the person
d. Being able to answer all the person's questions

3. Who should be trained to be an HIV counsellor?

a. Anyone who is interested in counselling and wants to help people
b. Only doctors
c. Only professional nurses
d. Only someone who is HIV positive themself

4. A characteristic of a good counsellor is:

a. To be kind, caring and understanding
b. To be firm and give clear advice
c. To be female and at least 40 years old
d. To have strong religious beliefs

5. What is the first step in providing counselling?

a. Giving answers to the person's problems
b. Taking action to solve the problems
c. Exploring the problems so that the person can understand which problems need to be tackled
d. Giving clear advice

6. The main aim of HIV counselling in pregnancy is:

a. To provide information and support the woman
b. To force the woman to change her behaviour
c. To persuade the woman to tell her husband the results of her HIV test
d. To teach the woman how to change her values

7. Counselling before an HIV test should be offered to pregnant women:

a. If the counsellor thinks the woman is at high risk of becoming infected with HIV
b. If the woman is not married
c. If the woman asks for counselling
d. Every time an HIV screening test is done

8. The decision to perform an HIV test should be taken by:

a. The hospital or clinic staff
b. The woman herself
c. The community
d. The pregnant woman's husband

9. What is an advantage of taking an HIV test?

a. If negative, the woman need not worry about safer sex practices
b. If negative, the woman can pay less for health insurance each month
c. If positive, the woman can make informed choices in her pregnancy
d. If positive, the doctors can arrange to have the infant adopted

10. What is a disadvantage of taking an HIV test?

a. The woman may be refused further antenatal care.
b. The woman may feel angry, afraid, depressed and despairing.
c. It is expensive and painful.
d. Dentists may refuse to treat her.

11. Who should be told the results of the HIV test?

a. The result should only be given to the woman's husband.
b. The result should be shared with all the women who were given counselling before the test.
c. The result should only be given to the employee.
d. The result should be given to the woman in private as soon as it becomes available.

12. What counselling should be given to a pregnant woman after a negative HIV result?

a. She should be told that she is unlikely to become HIV positive in future.
b. She should be encouraged to have as many infants as she wants as soon as possible while she is still HIV negative.
c. She should be counselled not to plan any further pregnancies.
d. She should be advised to practise safer sex.

13. When first telling a woman that she is HIV positive, the counsellor should:

a. Discuss safer sex with her
b. Allow her time to absorb the bad news and share her feelings

c. Encourage her not to worry about the being HIV positive as ARV drugs are available

d. Find out who infected her with HIV

14. What counselling is needed after a pregnant woman is informed that she has a positive HIV result?

a. She should be encouraged to identify her support system.

b. She should be told that she will eventually die of AIDS.

c. She should be given as much information about AIDS as possible.

d. She should be told not to have sexual intercourse with her partner.

15. What are common responses to being told that the HIV test is positive?

a. The woman immediately wants to inform her sexual partner.

b. The woman is relieved that her fear of having HIV infection has finally been confirmed.

c. The woman cannot believe the result and insists that there must be some mistake.

d. The woman accepts the information calmly with little emotional response.

16. How can a counsellor help a woman tell her sexual partner that she is HIV positive?

a. The woman should be encouraged to talk about her fear of telling her husband.

b. The midwife should tell the husband.

c. The husband should not be told at all.

d. The counsellor should tell the husband.

17. Who should an HIV-positive woman tell about her diagnosis?

a. She must tell her employer as this is required by law.

b. She must tell her partner immediately.

c. She should tell a trusted friend or family member who can support her.

d. She must tell her teacher if she is still at school.

18. How should an HIV-positive woman be counselled if she wants to fall pregnant?

a. Discuss why she wants to fall pregnant and explore what the effects would be for her and her infant if she fell pregnant.

b. Explain to her why she should not fall pregnant.

c. Encourage her to rather use a family planning method.

d. Help her to see that she is being selfish.

19. What advice about safer sex practices should be given to an HIV-positive woman?

a. She should not have sex.

b. She can have unprotected sex as she is already infected.

c. She should only have sex with HIV-positive men.

d. She should use condoms when having sex.

20. Healthcare workers who give HIV counseling:

a. Usually do not find counselling stressful.

b. Should only be allowed to counsel for six months as it is so stressful.

c. Should only be offered support and counselling themselves if they ask for it.

d. Should all have support and counselling to prevent burn out.

Answers

Test 1: Introduction to perinatal HIV

Question	Correct answer	Section
1.	a	1-2
2.	a	1-4
3.	c	1-6
4.	c	1-8
5.	b	1-12
6.	d	1-13
7.	d	1-14
8.	a	1-15
9.	b	1-16
10.	d	1-17
11.	c	1-20
12.	d	1-21
13.	a	1-23
14.	c	1-25
15.	c	1-26
16.	b	1-29
17.	c	1-30
18.	d	1-32
19.	a	1-34
20.	b	1-36

Test 2: HIV in pregnancy

Question	Correct answer	Section
1.	c	2-1
2.	d	2-3
3.	b	2-4
4.	a	2-5
5.	b	2-6
6.	c	2-8
7.	c	2-10
8.	b	2-12
9.	a	2-13
10.	c	2-16
11.	c	2-17
12.	c	2-17
13.	d	2-20
14.	a	2-21
15.	d	2-22
16.	a	2-23
17.	b	2–30
18.	d	2–32
19.	c	2-41
20.	b	2-48

Test 3: HIV during labour and delivery

Question	Correct answer	Section
1.	b	3-2
2.	a	3-3
3.	b	3-4
4.	d	3-5
5.	b	3-8
6.	a	3-9
7.	b	3-10
8.	a	3-11
9.	a	3-12
10.	c	3-14
11.	b	3-15
12.	d	3-16
13.	b	3-17
14.	c	3-19
15.	b	3-20
16.	b	3-22
17.	d	3-23
18.	c	3-25
19.	a	3-25
20.	c	3-29

Test 4: HIV in the newborn infant

Question	Correct answer	Section
1.	c	4-1
2.	d	4-2
3.	d	4-6
4.	a	4-7
5.	d	4-9
6.	a	4-14
7.	c	4-16
8.	a	4-17
9.	b	4-19
10.	c	4-20
11.	d	4-22
12.	b	4-23
13.	a	4-24
14.	c	4-25
15.	c	4-25
16.	a	4-34
17.	c	4-35
18.	b	4-37
19.	b	4-38
20.	d	4-40

Test 5: HIV and counselling

Question	Correct answer	Section
1.	c	5-1
2.	b	5-5
3.	a	5-6
4.	a	5-7
5.	c	5-11
6.	a	5-13
7.	d	5-16
8.	b	5-17
9.	c	5-20

10.	b	5-21	**16.**	a	5-26
11.	d	5-22	**17.**	c	5-27
12.	d	5-23	**18.**	a	5-31
13.	b	5-24	**19.**	d	5-35
14.	a	5-24	**20.**	d	5-38
15.	c	5-25			